W0105728

Metric Conversion Chart

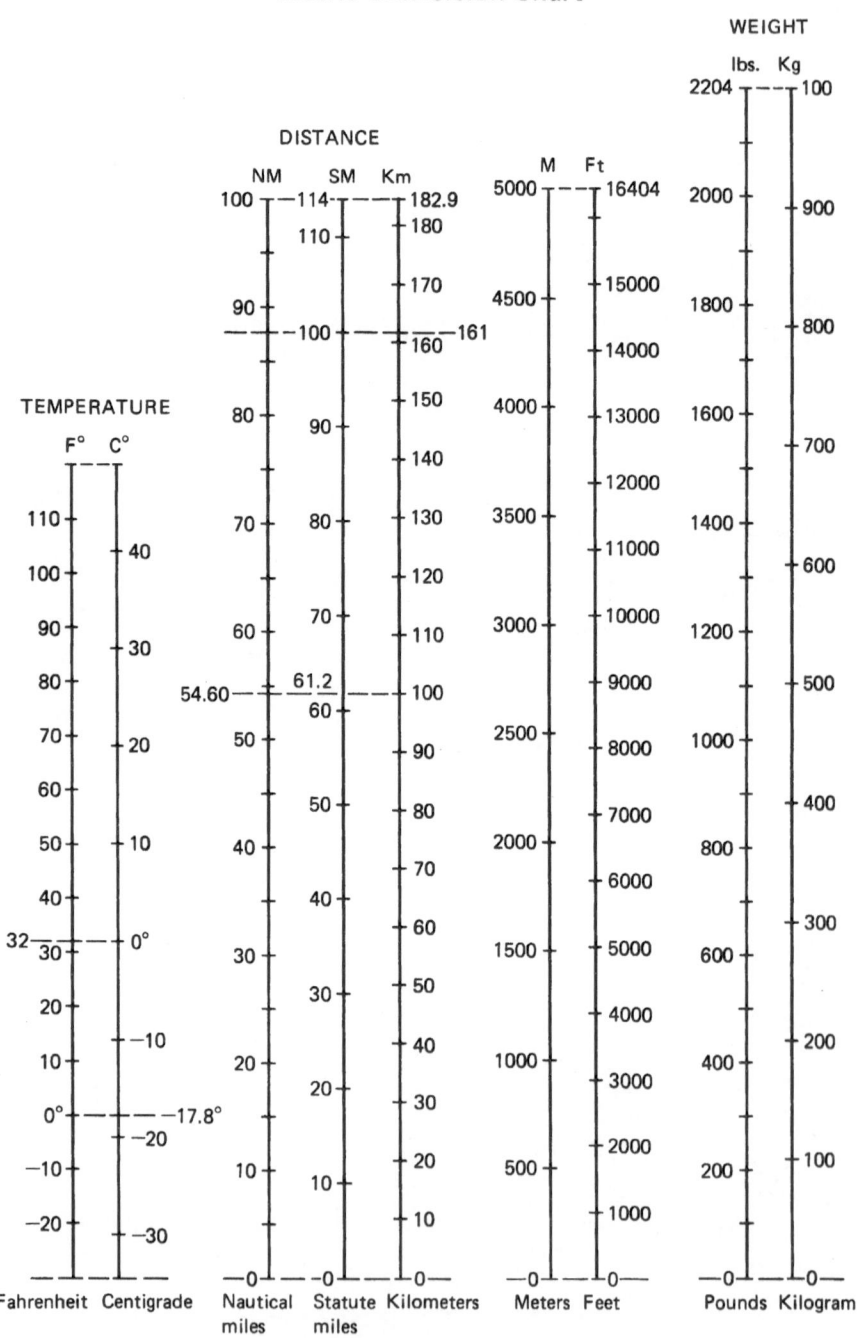

Airborne Care
of the Ill and Injured

Edward L. McNeil

Airborne Care
of the Ill and Injured

With 38 Illustrations

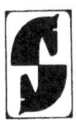

Springer-Verlag
New York Heidelberg Berlin

Edward L. McNeil, M.B., B.S., M.D.
Director
Department of Emergency Services
St. Agnes Hospital
White Plains, New York 10605, U.S.A.

Sponsoring Editor: Marie Low

Library of Congress Cataloging in Publication Data
McNeil, Edward L.
    Airborne care of the ill and injured.
    Includes index.
    1. Aviation medicine. 2. Airplane ambulances.
I. Title. [DNLM: 1. Aerospace medicine. 2. Aircraft.
3. Ambulances. 4. Emergency medical services.
5. Transportation of patients. WX 215 M478a]
RC1063.M36   1982   616.9'80213   82-19463

© 1983 by Springer-Verlag New York Inc.
All rights reserved. No part of this book may be translated or
reproduced in any form without written permission from
Springer-Verlag, 175 Fifth Avenue, New York, New York 10010, U.S.A.
The use of general descriptive names, trade names, trademarks, etc.,
in this publication, even if the former are not especially identified, is
not to be taken as a sign that such names, as understood by the Trade
Marks and Merchandise Marks Act, may accordingly be used freely by
anyone.

Typeset by Bi-Comp Incorporated, York, Pennsylvania

9 8 7 6 5 4 3 2 1

ISBN 978-1-4684-8681-0   ISBN 978-1-4684-8679-7 (eBook)
DOI 10. 1007/978-1-4684-8679-7

Contents

Foreword

From the unique position of a decade in government service, I was given the opportunity to observe the changes in the provision of emergency medical care across the country. In 1970, Emergency Medical Service (EMS) systems were a new and much needed development in the national health care delivery system. A systems approach to field casualty care has been progressively improved during each successive military conflict since the Civil War. These improvements were initiated after the medical care and evacuation disaster experienced by the Union Army of the Potomac at Bull Run on July 21, 1861. During the Civil War, major changes in administration, professional personnel, transportation, hospitals, sanitation, and medical records established patterns that have been continually refined and improved.

Stimulated by the pressing demands of war surgery and coupled with parallel advances in medical care over the last century, an almost unbelievable level of performance was realized in Vietnam. Advances in field resuscitation, efficiency of aeromedical transportation, and energetic treatment of military casualties have proved to be major factors in the decrease in death rates of battle casualties reaching facilities: from 8% in World War I to 4.5% in World War II to 2.5% in Korea and to less than 2% in Vietnam. As has been repeatedly demonstrated in previous military conflicts, the rapid aeromedical evacuation of the critically injured to adequately staffed and equipped advanced treatment (M.A.S.H.) units has shown that a highly perfected and well operated EMS system could also save lives in the civilian peacetime community.

The modern era of Emergency Medical Services (EMS) and the beginning of the civilian systems approach to improved emergency medical care was initiated in 1966 by the document, "Accidental Death and Disability—The Neglected Disease of Modern Society," prepared by the National Academy of Sciences, National Research Council. Among the basic building blocks and blueprints for improved emergency medical care programs outlined in this now-classic white paper, one specific recommendation relative to the regionalization of EMS was the "Initiation of pilot programs to evaluate automotive and helicopter ambulance services in sparsely populated areas and regions where many communities lack hospital facilities adequate to care for seriously injured persons."

Prehospital care now has a level of proficiency found only in small areas of the country 10 years ago, and it continues to improve. The capability to provide advanced life support (ALS) ranging from physician extenders (volunteers, emergency medical technicians, paramedics, nurses, and other designated providers) with essential medical control through sophisticated radio systems continues to expand.

In an EMS system, medical control provides the operational framework and justification for field paramedics and other physician extenders to provide emergency and interventive critical care treatments in out-of-hospital situations. It has been gratifying that so many physicians have come to realize that they have responsibility for the medical care of patients before they reach the hospital and are now more readily associated with those who provide that care.

A patient's illness or his injuries do not settle into a state of limbo during transport. The natural progression of acute disease and the pathophysiologic reactions to trauma continue and need to be assessed and ameliorated before a patient reaches the hospital. The organized utilization of aeromedical evacuation by both helicopter and fixed-wing vehicles further extends the "Golden Period" in which better resuscitation and definitive care can be made more readily available to the critically ill and injured.

Both autopsy and clinical studies have established "hard" mortality and morbidity statistics to make the argument for improved regional Trauma/EMS systems and the utilization of rapid air transportation services as a crucial aspect of these efforts.

The realization that there is a strong need for a systems approach to providing medical care for the patient transported by air is dawning, albeit tardily. More and more hospitals have built heliports and an increasing number of law enforcement personnel know how to clear an area to allow access or facilitate transfer. There is also an increasing interest in the use of conventional fixed-wing aircraft to extend the range of services to more distant areas.

Economics has prohibited reliance on dedicated air ambulances for the aeromedical transport of patients over moderate and long-range distances. Aircraft are still being used that are far from suitable for the safe transport of the ill and injured. The aviation environment presents many challenges to those attending patients who are in conditions especially susceptible to its vagaries. The basic underlying problems responsible for these challenges have not generally been recognized or adequately addressed. This book identifies those problems and provides sensible advice that should ensure safe and effective transfer by air that will not aggravate patients' illness or injury.

The past decade has seen incredible advances in the prehospital phase of our emergency medical system. The work with paramedic training, ambulance equipment and design, improved communication, transportation, and on-line medical control represents one of the finest chapters in the history of American medical achievements. This book represents a worthwhile and much needed addition to our collective progress in improving emergency medical services.

Dr. McNeil is one of the pioneers in the development of EMS. He has a perspective on all aspects of patient air transport. His experience in aeromedical transport abroad and in the U.S. has added to an even broader perspective on EMS. This book should broaden the interest of others involved in the care of patients during transport and instruct them on how to meet the challenges of the airborne care of the ill and injured.

David R. Boyd, M.D., C.M.
Maryland Institute for
    Emergency Medical Services
    Systems
Baltimore, Maryland

Preface

Less than 15 years ago, it tardily became apparent to the medical profession, and the public, that the care and transport of the sick and injured by the ambulance services was less than adequate. Since that time, enormous strides have been made improving the training and competency of those that man the ambulances and the ambulances are now better designed and equipped.

During the last few years, there has been a steady increase in the use of aircraft for the transport of patients. The majority of the missions flown are presently manned by medical personnel who are inadequately trained to care for patients in the aviation environment and are flown in aircraft that are either unsuitable or are not adequately equipped.

A significant number of aeromedical missions are transoceanic and expose a medical flight attendant to the medical environment of foreign countries where the language, customs, ethics, and the degree of medical sophistication are quite different from those of the flight attendant's home base. Such differences are to be found quite close to our shores and borders.

This book prepares medical technicians, nurses, and physicians in adapting their present skills and knowledge to the aviation environment and in giving some guidance on the conduct necessary to adjust to the circumstances found in other countries.

I am grateful that the National Highway Safety Administration of the U.S. Department of Transportation and the Commission on Emergency Medical Services of the American Medical Association have published "Air Ambulance Guidelines" (1981). These guidelines should stimulate interest in the aeromedical care of the ill and injured, especially the critically injured.

Acknowledgments

Numerous friends and colleagues in the aviation and the medical field have provided information which has helped in the writing of this manual. Some must be mentioned by name. Those not mentioned are not forgotten and are well appreciated for their assistance. Others who will remain nameless provided the experience, the satisfactions, and occasional fears. These are the patients who suffered my airborne care. To them this book is dedicated.

Two physicians in the United States who operate excellent air ambulance services are Wesley W. Bare, M.D. of North American Air Ambulance and Michael N. Cowan, M.D. of Air Ambulance, Inc., San Carlos, California. To both I express my gratitude for information gained from their experiences. I am also grateful to David Warburg of AI Ambulance in Mount Kisco, New York and formerly of SOS International Assistance. He first encouraged my entrance into the fascinating field of aeromedical evacuation.

I owe many thanks to Michael Wood, C.B.E., F.R.C.S., Chief of the Flying Doctor Service of East Africa and Peter Durner formerly of German Air Rescue for information and their encouragement. The United States Air Force has always been ready to answer questions and provide interesting and valuable information. For the reports on medical material items (USAF School of Aerospace Medicine), thanks are due for the assistance of Lt. Col. Robert E. Armstrong, USAF, Brooks AFD, Texas.

For information, documents, reports, and photographs regarding the operations of the Military Airlift Command aeromedical evacuation system, I thank Jack W. Jones, Lt. Col, USAF, MC, Chief, Aeromedical Evacuation Division, Office of the Command Surgeon, and Jacob T. Moll, Colonel, USAF, MC, Chief, Medical Readiness Division, Directorate of Medical Plans and Resources, Office of the Surgeon General.

Rudy Barnwell, respiratory therapist at the Northern Westchester Hospital Center, kindly assisted in clarifying certain points related to oxygen therapy.

Thanks are also due Dr. David Boyd for his encouragement and for kindly providing the foreword.

I am most grateful to Medicall International, a subsidiary of Credit-Card Services Corporation, Alexandria, Virginia, for permission to quote liberally from the manual for Flight Surgeons and Flight Nurses written by me when I was a consultant to that organization.

The following aircraft companies were kind enough to supply information and/or photographs:

Aerospatiale Helicopter Corporation
Atlantic Aviation
Beech Aircraft Corporation
Bell Helicopter Textron
British Aerospace Aircraft Group
Britten-Norman (Bembridge) Ltd.
Canadair
Cessna Aircraft Company

Consolidated Aircraft
Construccionees Aeronauticas, S.A.
Dassault International
Fairchild Swearingen Aviation Corp.
Falcon Jet Corporation
Gates Learjet Corporation
Gulfstream American
Hughes Helicopters, Inc.
Lockheed Corporation
Messerschmitt-Boelkow-Blohm
Piper Aircraft Corporation
Rockwell International
Short Brothers Ltd.

Finally, thanks are also due the staff of Springer-Verlag, especially Marie Low, Larry Meyer, and Bill Gabello.

1

THE ATTENDANT
AND HIS ENVIRONMENT

THE MEDICAL FLIGHT ATTENDANT

This text is intended to provide sufficient practical information regarding the physiological and technical aspects of air transport of patients so that a physician who is familiar with its contents will be able to give sound, practical advice to air ambulance operators, regardless of whether or not the physician has ever flown as a medical flight attendant. More importantly, this book was written for and directed at those physicians, nurses, and allied health professionals who are directly responsible for the medical transfer of patients by aircraft. These responsibilities are varied: from clinical care that requires thoughtful modification of methods that might be applied in a hospital, to coordination of multiple transfer stages, to diplomacy abroad, to the enhancement of an exciting aspect of emergency medical services.

Fitness of the Medical Flight Attendant

To meet the varied responsibilities and to cope with the unusual circumstances that may occur, especially on international flights, physical and mental fitness is essential. Physicians, nurses, and ambulance captains who are used to standing back and watching others use their strength to lift patients may be surprised to find, on their first flight as an attendant, that they must now use their own muscular strength. Rarely are there enough strong hands to permit the medical flight attendant the luxury of being a spectator. Loading and unloading a patient on a stretcher into and out of an aircraft necessitates lifting at heights and angles that are not encountered in ground ambulance work.

The flight attendant should have no disabilities that might hinder the performance of his duties in the aviation environment, whether these disabilities are of a chronic nature or are simply temporary illnesses or injuries. Individuals with hypertension, pulmonary deficiencies, anemia, or other chronic illnesses that would be aggravated by flying should disqualify themselves from aeromedical duties. A physical examination should be taken during the year prior to flying to learn whether any chronic illnesses exist or whether other contraindications to flight duty are present.

Weight
Excess body weight is known to be associated with other physical disorders that might disqualify an individual from flight duties. Weight is also important with regard to payload restrictions in small, light aircraft; stresses on parts of the aircraft; and balance of the aircraft with movements within the cabin.

Height
The configurations of the doors, the cabin headroom, and the seating arrangements in small aircraft make excessive height something of a problem, but less of a problem than excessive weight.

Motion Sickness

A medical flight attendant may be the right size and weight and may be in perfect physical and mental health, but is prone to motion sickness. Flights are coordinated to try to avoid turbulent air conditions whenever possible, but some degree of disturbing motion must be anticipated in all types of aircraft. At times turbulence can be so severe that even a veteran with the most stable vestibular apparatus and the strongest stomach will experience motion sickness. Prospective medical flight attendants should therefore have no contraindications to the taking of antiemetic medication.

Upper Respiratory Infection (URI)

Acute respiratory infections are not only potentially damaging to patients under care and to other members of the crew, but they can also present the hazards associated with blocked sinus ostia and eustachian tubes. The ventilation systems of some aircraft are such that airborne disease organisms can be circulated repeatedly, and the next users of the plane may be at risk.

Immunizations

Those whose duties may take them to countries where serious endemic diseases exist should be up to date with immunizations that are properly recorded on a World Health Organization immunization record. This record should be carried with a valid passport (see International Travel).

Drugs and Alcohol

Companies that operate aircraft must follow regulations that impose restrictions on air crew regarding the taking of medications and the ingestion of alcohol in the hours prior to flight duty. These restrictions vary slightly from country to country and are based on studies that positively relate deterioration in performance of duties to blood alcohol and drug levels. Elements in the nature of flying can hasten the onset of fatigue (mental and physical); certain drugs and alcohol most definitely compound this problem.

Medical flight crews, especially when attending critically ill or injured patients, are under as much (or more) stress as the flight deck crew. The medical member of the crew may have to perform considerably more physical work than those in the cockpit.

An air ambulance company that regularly engages medical flight attendants should have sensible company regulations that restrict the performance of duties within an appropriate number of hours following alcohol ingestion.

Contact Lenses

The wearing of contact lenses is not recommended in the aviation environment except on short missions as a medical flight attendant. Corrective lenses in frames should be available for immediate use in the event that the corneal lenses require removal.

Appearance and Conduct

Those attending the sick and injured on aeromedical missions should present themselves to patients, clients, and other personnel as clean and groomed professionals. Hairstyles and fingernails should not interfere with attending the patient or using equipment. Long hair should be tied back and fingernails should be short.

Dress should be practical. A jumpsuit or slacks covered with a jacket or shirt having an adequate number of pockets is suitable. All items of clothing should be in professional colors.

Dress should also bear some insignia which announces that the wearer is a medical officer. A light-colored bushjacket is ideal and may assist in gaining attention and respect when meeting officials of other countries at airport checkpoints and at medical facilities.

High heels and open-toed sandals are hazardous during duty on board aircraft. Tobacco breath, alcohol breath, perfume, and aftershave lotions are upsetting to an ill or injured person. Breath fresheners may be appropriate before going on duty.

Conduct Abroad

At times a medical flight attendant may have to assess the condition and needs of a patient in a foreign hospital or somewhere other than home base where the standards of medical care and the facilities are not up to the standards to which he is accustomed. In the majority of such places the staff is practicing under those conditions because of a shortage of space, equipment, or adequate training. A visiting medical flight attendant should refrain from criticism and should be careful to avoid derogatory remarks. Whenever possible, appreciation should be shown for what has already been done for the patient with the limited resources available. The cooperation resulting from this attitude can be extremely beneficial to both the attendant and the patient.

Qualifications of Medical Flight Attendants

On short flights within a country, where the patient has minor injuries or a stable illness of minimal seriousness, the basic competency required to transport a patient by ground vehicle plus the general principles of aviation medicine may be sufficient. On longer flights, especially those that are transoceanic, or where the patient has a more serious illness or injury, a considerable degree of specialized knowledge may be required to accept and act on the medical responsibilities that may present themselves. Courses of instruction are now given to impart this specialized knowledge. It is hoped that in the near future there will be a way of identifying

those physicians, nurses, and paramedics who have had such training
and have demonstrated their competency.

Physicians

Medical flight crew candidates should be chosen from those who have
extensive experience in critical care, including advanced cardiac life
support. Physicians must be in active medical practice and must be licensed to practice medicine in the state or country in which they reside.
Experienced emergency physicians and casualty officers usually have
the necessary breadth of knowledge and experience to make them suitable for extracurricular flying duties, provided that they are physically
and mentally fit after their regular work. Emergency physicians can also
alter their working schedules more easily than other specialists or gener-
alists in order to make themselves available for duties that might extend
over a few days or longer.

Nurses

Nurses must also be licensed and registered in the state or country in
which they reside. They should have received training in critical care
nursing and have had considerable experience in critical care units or in
emergency departments in which critical care is provided. The ability to
assess a patient's condition with regard to all systems is desirable. A
flight nurse should be familiar with the techniques and equipment used
for respiratory assistance, airway clearance, chest tube care and connection, orthopedic traction, cardiac monitoring, and intravenous therapy.

A nurse must be prepared to make medical decisions when necessary
within the limits of any protocols in force. Standing orders should be
available to the flight nurse, and radio communication with a directing
physician should be made where circumstances dictate and permit (see
Communications).

Medical Technicians, Paramedics, and Respiratory Therapists

When members of this group of medical personnel perform duties as
medical flight attendants, they should know who is the physician directing the medical aspects of the mission; each should be conversant with
the other's abilities and responsibilities. Medical technicians must be
certified or licensed in the state or country in which they reside.

Transport of "Care-to-Patient" Mission

There will be times when a patient who is critically injured or ill cannot
be moved until specialist care has arrived. A team may need to be flown
in with the necessary equipment to give advanced medical or surgical
care. If there is any chance that the patient will return with the team by
plane, a trained medical flight attendant should be part of that team so
that he can advise on the aeromedical aspects of preflight preparation
and care during transport.

THE AVIATION ENVIRONMENT

Physics

Physics, as applicable to patient care in the aviation environment, refers to the confines, conformations, and mechanical capabilities of the aircraft, on the ground as well as in the air. The physical capabilities of the aircraft to accelerate, take off, fly, gain altitude, maneuver, descend, land, and decelerate all have influences on the physiology of those on board: patient, flight crew, and medical flight attendant alike.

Physiology

The influences on physiology have a direct relationship to the physics of mechanical inertia, gravity, and the pressure and temperature changes associated with alteration of altitude. There are also influences on acoustics and optics.

Physical and Physiological Considerations in Aeromedical Transport

Important considerations must be given when transporting a patient by air that are usually not given when transporting by ground ambulance. Some of these considerations are:

1. Sudden movement in *any* direction.
2. Accelerating and decelerating forces sufficient to redistribute the body fluids.
3. Gas expansion or contraction with changes in cabin atmospheric pressure (within the body or within equipment).
4. Temperature changes may be more extreme and more rapid.
5. Increase in visual stimuli.
6. Wider range and intensity of acoustic stimuli.
7. Wider range of olfactory stimuli.

Depending upon the type of aircraft being utilized as an air ambulance, additional considerations include:

8. Limitation of dimensions of access and available cabin space.
9. Difficulties associated with maneuvering a stretcher patient through a confining door that is not at normal level.
10. Limitations of payload.
11. Restrictions related to the center of gravity of the aircraft (in flight and when the plane is resting on its undercarriage).
12. Limitations on amount and type of equipment that can be powered by the electrical system.
13. Limitations on levels of electromagnetic interference produced by carried medical equipment (navigational equipment may be sensitive).
14. Length of time on board without relief for replenishing supplies and attending to excretory functions.

15. Loss of electrical power when engines are shut down, with consequent loss of cabin heat or cabin cooling.
16. Jet or propeller streams and rotating blades.
17. Vibration.
18. Wider variety of size and type of vehicle when compared to ground ambulances.
19. Varied stimuli provocative of "excitement" (in the patient *and* in the medical flight attendant).

Each of the preceding points will be covered in some detail under specific section headings, as will the modifications in medical care necessitated by the aviation environment. It should be remembered that the aviation environment has influences on the efficiency of certain types of medical equipment, especially those aiding respiration, as well as on the physiologic functioning of the patient and the crew.

Because modern air travel is relatively comfortable, it is widely believed that pressurized aircraft are capable of maintaining the cabin atmospheric pressure at the pressure normally experienced on the ground. The "ear popping" is believed to be due to some slight delays in pressurization. This is a belief which is not justified by the facts. It has led to medical problems in numerous patients and even to deaths.

It is advantageous for aircraft to fly at high altitudes for reasons of speed, fuel economy, and lack of turbulence. Most long-distance airline flights are at altitudes of between 30,000 and 40,000 feet. Some of the smaller jet aircraft (such as the Gates Lear) are most economically flown at 41,000 feet. The degree of pressurization allowable in the cabin of an aircraft is strictly limited by the structural strength of its fuselage at its weakest point. The fuselage in this context must include doors, ports, and windows. If the limit is exceeded, the fuselage will burst. The strength to withstand the pressure differences between the inside and outside of the fuselage is controlled by the strength/weight ratios of the various parts of the fuselage.

These facts mean that the pressure within the cabin of an airliner at cruising height is equivalent to that found at 5000 to 8000 feet of altitude, 6000 feet now being (supposedly) the minimum cabin pressure equivalent allowable.

Two concerns dominate the modifications necessary in medical care when altitude is gained:

1. The partial pressure of oxygen available to the alveolar sacs of the lungs diminishes to a significant degree. Unless this is compensated for in some way, hypoxemia can ensue.
2. Gas which is trapped in body cavities or in medical equipment, such as intravenous fluid containers and suction bottles, expands to a significant degree. (Of equal importance is the fact that gas contracts as altitude is lost.)

The above concerns can be partly overcome by flying at low altitudes where the cabin pressure remains near that of the ground. However, low-altitude flying has severe disadvantages. Air turbulence is most prevalent at low altitudes and can be severe enough to prevent proper medical care from being given to a patient. Adverse weather conditions are more often encountered nearer the ground. Other disadvantages are the diminished safety from navigational hazards (natural and man-made, including other aircraft) and diminished performance of the craft (speed and fuel consumption). Prolonged passage through turbulent air is also a strain on the plane.

On balance, it is far more beneficial for a patient to be flown at high altitudes in a pressurized aircraft when any transfer of considerable distance is undertaken. The effects of reduced oxygen and the expansion of gases can be countered by the application of various medical methods.

Although a medical transfer flight may have a high cruising altitude, the plane must climb and descend through the lower altitude zones where uncomfortable turbulence exists. The methods of securing the patient, equipment, and the medical flight attendant are therefore of great importance. Sudden movements can occur in *any* direction and be of considerable severity. The author has experienced a sudden and unexpected drop of over 1000 feet in a large aircraft. Fortunately, this type of experience is rare.

Reassurances are in order for those who are new to flying, especially in light aircraft. Danger usually follows only from low degrees of competence on the part of those who maintain and fly the aircraft. In general, however, the competence of aircraft pilots and servicing mechanics exceeds that of personnel maintaining and driving ground transport vehicles. There is generous overcompensation of care to prevent accidents, and the certifying authorities of most countries have strict requirements regarding the fitness and abilities of those who fly, navigate, operate, and maintain aircraft.

Altitude and movement are not the only factors influencing the care of patients in the aviation environment. Noise generated by engines, wind and air movement, and motors of many sorts (inside and outside the cabin) must be taken into account. The visual fields must tolerate light from strange directions, of differing qualities, and endowed with unusual movements.

Although the dangers of flying are more imagined than real, some risks attending medical evacuation are real and not very apparent. One of these dangers relates to the transfer of diseases and disease vectors during international travel. Information will be provided later in this book to minimize these dangers.

DUTIES TO THE PATIENT

It might seem superfluous to mention certain basic tenets of patient care that are normally concerns of all medical personnel wherever they practice their art. However, they are worth reinforcing because aeromedical care is practiced in an environment full of distractions. These distractions can hamper logical thought at a time when special attention must be paid to facets of medical care that assume added importance in the aviation environment.

The excitement of flying derives not only from the experience of flight itself but also from the visual stimuli associated with it: in the airport, on the ramp or apron, inside and outside the aircraft. There are lights of many sorts and a variety of noises and vibrations not usually present at bedside. There are bodily sensations related to movement, acceleration, and deceleration. Air is moving in and out of body cavities. There is a "circus" in the vestibular apparatus. The patient, too, reacts differently to his illness or injuries because of both the psychological effects of his predicament and the alteration of symptoms provoked by the vagaries of the aviation environment.

A checklist of the major duties toward a patient can give logical direction to medical care in the air. These duties can be analyzed from the patient's and from the attendant's point of view. From the medical flight attendant's point of view, the key elements are *safety* and *comfort*.

Safety

The patient must be made as safe as possible:

Within the physical environment:
1. Safety from undue movement
2. Safety from harmful extremes of temperature and pressure
3. Safety from harmful noise levels and intense light
4. Safety from toxic, ignitable, or explosive fumes
5. Safety from harmful radiation

As regards medical integrity:
1. Safe circulatory volume
2. Safe oxygen-carrying capacity of the blood
3. Circulatory efficiency—rate, rhythm, and cardiac power
4. Adequate oxygenation and ventilation
5. Safe fluid balance—intake and output
6. Safe electrolyte balance
7. Protection from, or counteraction of, the harmful effects of drugs

Comfort

The patient must be made as comfortable as possible:

1. Physically
2. Mentally

Consideration of the patient's point of view can guide the medical flight attendant to other duties. Those duties, in order of importance to the patient, cover (1) breathing; (2) pain; (3) fear; (4) thirst; (5) elimination; (6) general physical comfort; and (7) hunger.

Breathing

To the patient, the ability to breathe adequately is of paramount importance.

Duty. Ensure that the airway is as unobstructed as possible; that ventilatory capacity is not lessened by mechanical hindrances to respiratory effort; that adequate oxygenation is provided; and that as changes occur in the physiological environment, they are compensated for. Respiratory equipment that may be needed by the patient must be available and in good condition. Enough oxygen to meet the patient's needs and last the length of the flight must be on board.

Pain

Consideration must be given to the deleterious effects of severe pain on the autonomic nervous system, and to its association with endocrine secretions. The excretion of catecholamines, occurring with injury and pain, can increase certain tissue oxygen requirements and aggravate cellular damage. Pain can also disrupt clear cerebral functioning, making rapport between the patient and the attendant difficult and clouding the patient's interpretations of his sensory experiences and needs.

Duty. To prevent, relieve, or minimize pain by physical or pharmacologic means. The physical means might include the application of cold or warm compresses, massage, or the alteration of posture. The medical flight attendant must have available a variety of oral and systemic analgesics.

Fear

Although many people have flown in large commercial airliners, not many have experienced flying in smaller, light aircraft that are more troubled by turbulent air conditions. The lesser weight and speed of small aircraft make them respond more uncomfortably to turbulent air. Many of them do not have the capability of flying at altitudes above the level of which the worst turbulence is found.

A bouncing environment can be a source of fear, especially to one who is ill or injured. A patient may be fearful of a morbid outcome of his medical condition that necessitated his evacuation by air. Whatever the source of fear, it can have harmful physiological effects similar, in some respects, to those provoked by pain. Tachycardia with elevated blood pressure can occur. In some patients there may be a vagal reaction, with lowering of blood pressure or syncope. Diaphoresis can be severe, with fluid loss and overcooling.

Duty. To communicate an air of professional confidence through calmness and reassurance, and by giving valid explanations to the patient of what he is experiencing or might experience. Everything possible should be done to minimize aggravating experiences which might provoke fear. Preflight sedation can diminish fear and its effects. In appropriate cases, preflight tranquilization might be necessary. A good bedside (or stretcherside) manner can do much to alleviate fear. In this respect, the importance of hands-on care should be mentioned. Communication by touch can afford much reassurance. There are many opportunities to provide true hands-on care. A patient should never be connected to the person attending him solely by a stethoscope. The free hand can hold the patient firmly by the shoulder or hand or be placed on the patient's forehead.

Thirst

Thirst is not only an aggravating symptom to the patient, but it can also be an important symptom indicating a problem in fluid balance and should always be taken seriously by the medical flight attendant. If the symptom of thirst is related to medication (e.g., Compazine), an explanation should be given to the patient as to why he feels thirsty, and other methods must be used to assess fluid needs.

Duty. To have the necessary fluids available and provide them as needed in the most palatable form in keeping with the medical needs or restrictions of the patient. If intravenous therapy is indicated, the intravenous line should be started before the plane is in flight and before undue movement adds difficulty to the venipuncture technique. Intravenous lines must be protected from tangling or compression, the flow monitored frequently, and care taken to prevent air embolus during the rise of cabin altitude.

Elimination

When there is an urge to urinate or defecate, extreme discomfort can occur if the means of relief are not immediately available.

Duty. Preflight attendance to these functions can alleviate many in-flight problems. Even on short flights, the necessary equipment should be available. On longer flights, when bedpans and urinals are almost sure to be required, sanitary, leak-proof storage bags must be available if conventional airline toilets are not on board.

General Physical Comfort

There are many ways physical comfort may be compromised on an air ambulance stretcher. It is very important that the patient be secured against the consequences of sudden vertical movement and during acceleration and deceleration. The straps and buckles can be prudently placed and padded where necessary. The head can be raised or lowered and well-supported as the patient's condition allows. The most common causes of discomfort are lying on buckles or pieces of equipment and pressure against the safety rails. Care should be taken to ensure that safety straps are not too tight and do not restrict respiratory movements of the thorax or abdomen. A patient with compromised pulmonary function may require all the movement of the thoracic cage and diaphragm that he can muster in order to provide an adequate vital capacity for his respiratory needs.

Duty. To provide a conscious effort to safely reduce or prevent discomfort for the patient. The means of relieving the discomfort caused by barotitis of the sinuses and middle ear will be discussed elsewhere, as will the methods of diminishing and treating airsickness.

Hunger

Good preflight planning and preparation can take care of any nutritional needs of the patient on long-distance transfers. If food needs to be provided in flight, a sensible choice of packed foods should be made, taking into account any preferences of the patient. A thermos or two of different warm and cold beverages can give pleasure, nutrition, and can meet necessary fluid needs.

Duty. Plan and prepare to meet the nutritional needs of the patient. This is best done at the point of origin of the patient transfer or by arrangement with the flight crew. You will find the experienced pilot very versatile at procuring food and drink out of the blue at stopovers in strange airports.

Further Duties

Other duties of the medical flight attendant indirectly provide important services for the patient and those others who may be accompanying him.

Flight Crew Liaison

It is important that there be full cooperation between pilot and attendant in modifying flight maneuvers according to the condition of the patient. Before any flight, there should be a discussion with the pilot regarding the means and methods of air to ground radio communications. Discussions with the flight crew can allow for suitable compromises with regard to flight maneuvers, altitude, cabin pressure and temperature, and lengths of hops and stopovers.

A medical flight attendant should make himself aware of the capabilities of the aircraft to be used for the patient transfer. These include its cruising speed and range, optimum operating altitude and pressurization efficiency, fuel reserves, payload, and oxygen and electrical supplies.

Preflight and inflight liaison with the pilot can make joint decisions easier to arrive at should they need to be made regarding whether to abort a transfer, turn back, or make an emergency landing somewhere other than at the predetermined airport.

The Environment

The importance of the physiologic changes that can occur with changes in the aviation environment make it a duty of the medical flight attendant to know and to be able to predict the barometric pressure in the cabin. It is usually inconvenient for a pilot or copilot to give a running commentary on what the cabin's relative altitude is or will be. It can also be annoying for the medical flight attendant to be constantly asking for this information. These difficulties can be overcome by the medical flight attendant having an altimeter as part of his own equipment (Fig. 1). A light and cheap instrument can indicate the cabin altitude to within 200 feet, which is adequate for the purposes intended. The author uses

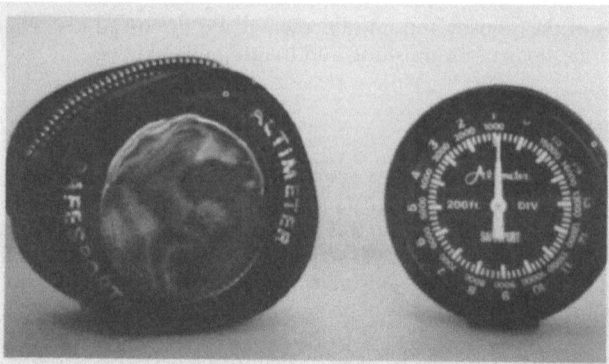

Figure 1. Pocket altimeter and carrying case. Diameter 2.5 inches. Weight 3 oz.

Model A1400 from the Safesport Manufacturing Company, Denver, Colorado 80202. It costs approximately $16 and was designed for use by mountaineers.

Documentation
It is the duty of the medical flight attendant to keep adequate records and to complete a mission report so that necessary medical records bridge those from the origin of transfer and those of the receiving facility.

THE COCKPIT CREW

The importance of liaison with the cockpit crew has already been touched on.

Before a flight, the pilot will have obtained certain information from A.T.C. (Air Traffic Control) and from the flight coordinator regarding weather conditions and air turbulence along the intended route of the flight. The prevailing weather conditions at the destination will be known, as will be the E.T.A. (estimated time of arrival). This information should be passed on to the medical flight attendant in order that it may be taken into account in the care of the patient.

The limitations placed on continuous flying hours for air crew and specified rest periods between flights may cause some stopovers or turn-arounds to be longer than anticipated. In such cases, arrangements may have to be made to transfer the patient to a suitable facility during the delay. Emergency departments of hospitals are usually cooperative in this respect and they can be used if near enough to the airstrip and proper ground transport is available. A pilot will usually know what space might be available within the airport facilities, or he can ascertain this information by radio before landing.

When Not to Distract the Cockpit Crew

On longer flights, a copilot may be on board and will be able to answer the questions of the medical flight attendant without distracting the pilot from his duties. However, during landing and takeoff, both the pilot and the copilot need to give their full attention to the control of the aircraft and should not be distracted.

Runway Conditions

A good pilot will give the medical flight attendant any warnings that are appropriate when runway conditions are such that a landing may be expected to have unusual characteristics.

In some underdeveloped countries and even in some out of the way places elsewhere, the condition of the runway and its length will have to be determined by the pilot. A short runway may call for more severe braking and, on rare occasions, for a spin stop (swinging the plane around suddenly). Crosswind landings on small airstrips may necessitate making sudden changes in direction and wing angulation. The runway may not be smooth, and a rough landing may be expected.

Where there is no tarmac surface, the Royal Flying Doctor Service of Australia checks out the surface condition of an airstrip by driving a motor vehicle over it before a plane lands.

There can be anxiety for the patient and his attendant should more than one pass need to be made over the airstrip before eventually landing. The pilot may have to chase cattle, wild animals, or people off the strip before it is clear to land. If the medical attendant can be informed of what to expect during an unusual landing and he can relay this information in a tactful way to the patient, discomfort and fright can be minimized.

Camaraderie

Any difficulties, discomforts, or apprehensions suffered during a flight are most often compensated for by the camaraderie to be enjoyed with the cockpit crew. The medical flight attendant should attempt to convey to the patient that he is included in this camaraderie. A good pilot of an air ambulance will always make himself known to the patient and offer words aimed at reassuring him and communicating concern.

2

REGULATIONS AND OPERATIONS

THE AIR AMBULANCE

There are air ambulance companies that are solely dedicated to air ambulance work. Their aircraft are permanently equipped to carry patients and are modified in ways to improve their ability to meet this function. However, because of cost factors, such aircraft are usually of a type that have limitations of performance with regard to range and speed that make their use for transfers over 1000 miles unsuitable. This is overcome by using, on a charter basis, aircraft that are faster, have greater range, and are more sophisticated. Since very few of these very expensive planes are structured for aeromedical use, they have to be modified as the need arises. There is a remarkable choice of aircraft that might be used to transport patients.

What is intriguing is that most aircraft that have been chosen to be used as air ambulances give the impression that they were chosen for their aesthetic appearance. It could be argued that the adaptability of an aircraft to ambulance work is inversely proportional to the degree of its elegance.

Ground ambulances have gone through a similar phase in the United States. It is only relatively recently that the sleek, shiny, hearse-like vehicles have been replaced by box-like units mounted on truck chassis or by units resembling bakery vans, with practical improvements. The changes have been in both the patients' and the attendants' interest.

There are aircraft that could win prizes for ugliness. Some of these have attributes which make them very suitable for air ambulance work over short and medium ranges. Many of them are S.T.O.L. aircraft (short takeoff and landing), which means that they can utilize very small airstrips. Some of them have unexpected speed and range.

The *Short Skyvan 3M* is an example of a useful "ugly" (Fig. 2). It can economically cruise at about 200 miles per hour and can takeoff and land in less than 800 feet. Its long range is 950 miles. Over a shorter range it can carry a payload up to 5000 lbs. Large doors at the rear make for easy loading; they are 6 feet 6 inches high and 6 feet 5 inches wide. There is 18 feet of usable cabin length.

Another aircraft that does not look like the more conventional air ambulance is the *201 Arava* made by Israel Aircraft Industries (Fig. 3). It also has excellent access at the rear by the cone-shaped aft part of the cabin swinging to the right. It has S.T.O.L. capabilities and can takeoff and land in less than 800 feet. Cruising speed with a payload expected for an aeromedical flight is approximately 200 miles per hour, with a range of 800 miles. It has been used to carry 12 patients on stretchers and 2 medical attendants (not recommended), which gives some indication of the space available and the load it can carry. It can reach an altitude of 25,000 feet.

Most of the S.T.O.L. aircraft are unable to fly at high altitudes and are therefore unable to take advantage of the calmer air above 25,000 feet. However, their use should be considered for short- and medium-range flights of up to 800 miles. Some can carry as many as 18 passengers and larger payloads, allowing the transport of multiple patients, an adequate number of medical attendants, and heavier medical equipment. It is this

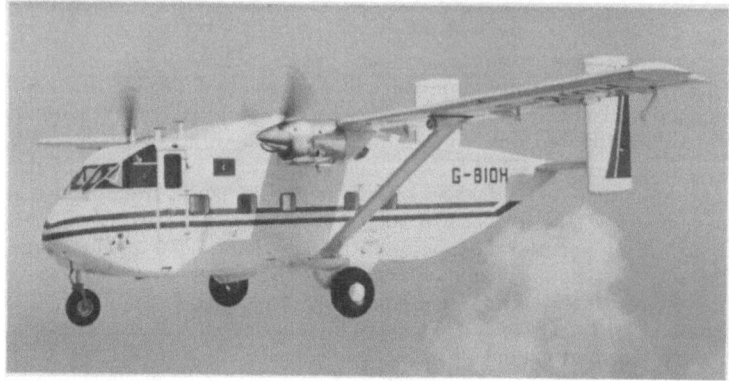

A

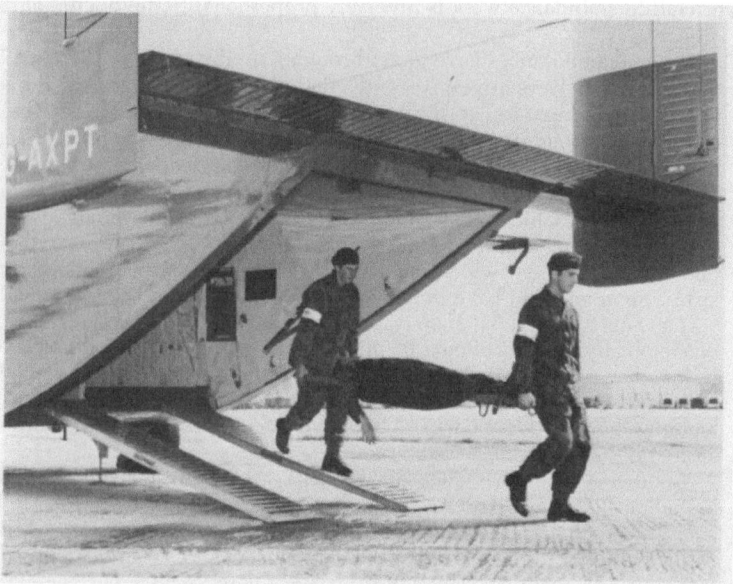

B

Figure 2. A–C: Skyvan 3M. Turboprop S.T.O.L. aircraft with rear ramp loading. For mass evacuations, it can accommodate 12 stretchers. It can be used on unpaved airstrips. Noise and vibration levels are high in the utility model because of its unlimited square sides. For aeromedical work, noise insulation is required. (Courtesy of Short Brothers Limited, Belfast, North Ireland.)

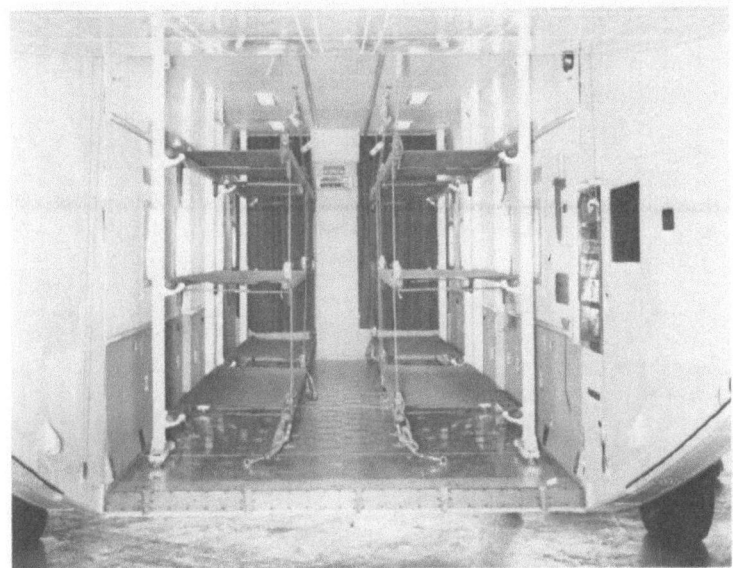

Figure 2C.

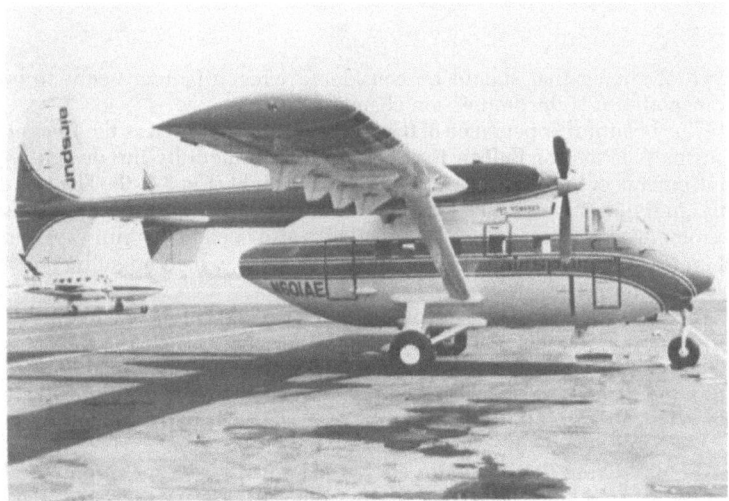

Figure 3. 201 Arava. Israel Aircraft Industries. It can be used on very short runways. (Courtesy of Consolidated Aircraft Corporation, Dania, Florida.)

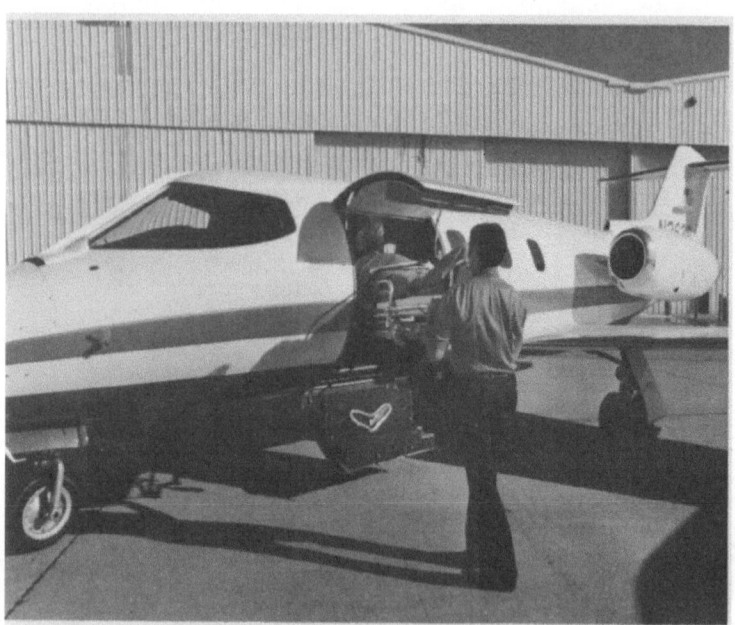

Figure 4. Gates Learjet 25. Note the size of the door and that the steps are incorporated into the door. Also note the height of the stretcher must be lifted for loading. (Courtesy of Gates Learjet Corporation, Tucson, Arizona.)

type of aircraft that should be considered when a patient needs to be transported in a decompression chamber.

The beautiful appearance of the smaller jet aircraft such as the Learjet, Cessna Citation, or Falcon is almost forced on them by the design requirements of high-speed and high-altitude flight (Figs. 4–9). The same design requirements make for limited but workable cabin space as far as aeromedical use is concerned. Such planes also need longer runways and therefore cannot use many of the smaller airstrips which might be much closer to hospitals.

To maintain the integrity of the fuselage with high inside-outside pressure differentials and to maintain the aerodynamic shape, the doors of these fast jets have to be relatively small. Steps are often incorporated into the doors. Larger doors would add too much uneven weight. Wide doors can also limit the placement of passenger seats in the limited cabin space.

Before giving the details of aircraft commonly used for aeromedical transport, it should be useful to consider the primary and secondary characteristics of aircraft so that an impression may be gained of their adaptability to specific aeromedical needs. These needs vary in definite ways according to the medical needs of the patient, where he is to be

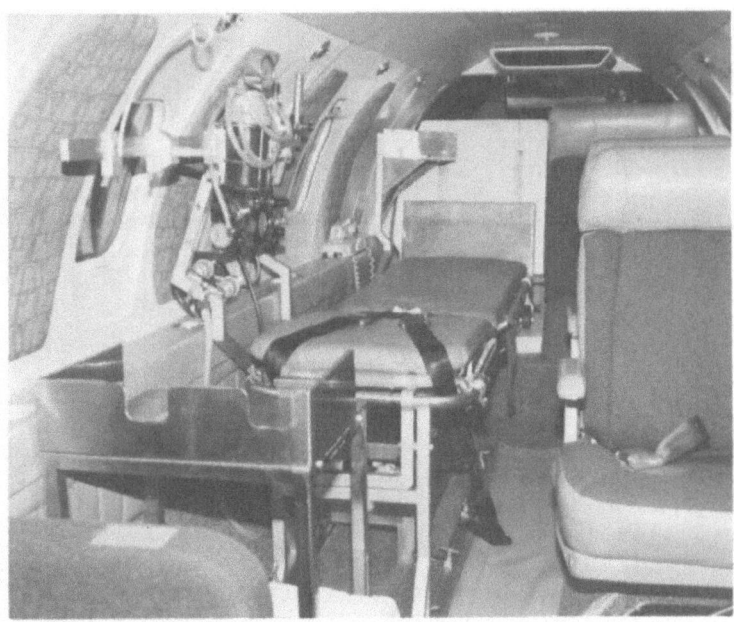

Figure 5. The interior of the Learjet 25, modified as an air ambulance. (Courtesy of Gates Learjet Corporation, Tucson, Arizona.)

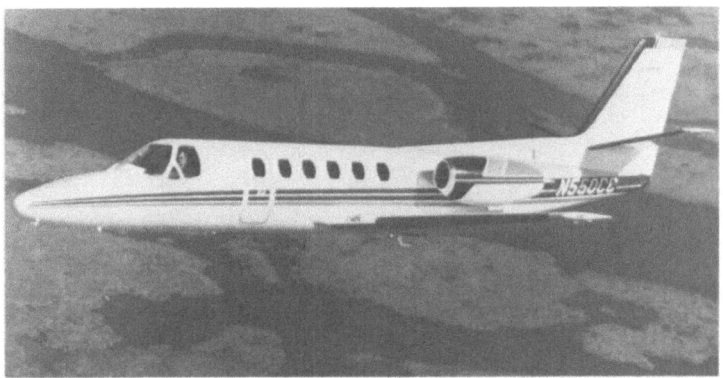

Figure 6. Cessna Citation II. Cruising speed of 380 miles per hour; has range of 2000 miles. Runway requirement is 2400 feet. (Courtesy of Cessna Aircraft Company, Wichita, Kansas.)

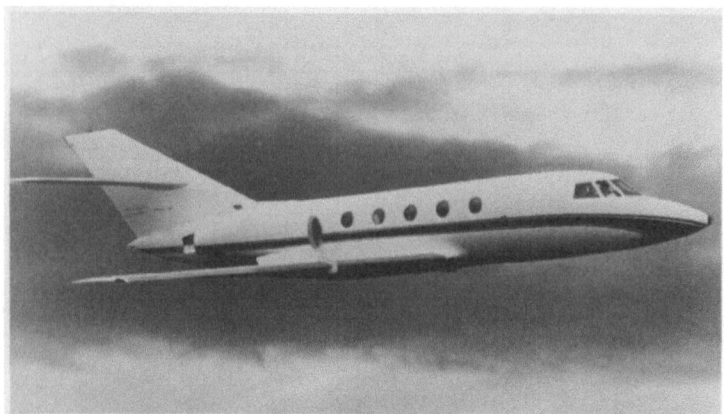

Figure 7. Falcon 20. Avions Marcel Dassault-Breguet Aviation. It is used as an air ambulance in France. The cabin can be maintained at sea level pressure at altitudes up to 23,000 feet. (Courtesy of Dassault International, Vaucresson, France.)

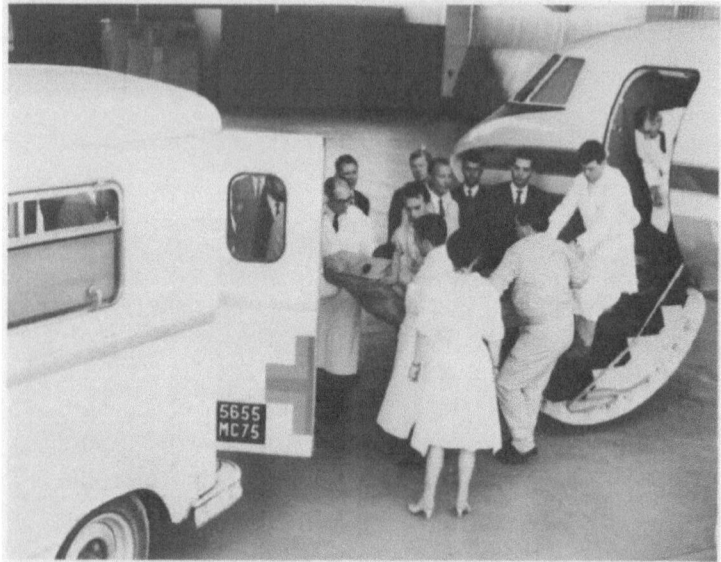

Figure 8. Loading a patient into a Falcon 50. Note the door size, that the steps are part of the door, and the stop wires supporting the steps. A vacuum mattress is being used as a stretcher. (Courtesy of Dassault International, Vaucresson, France.)

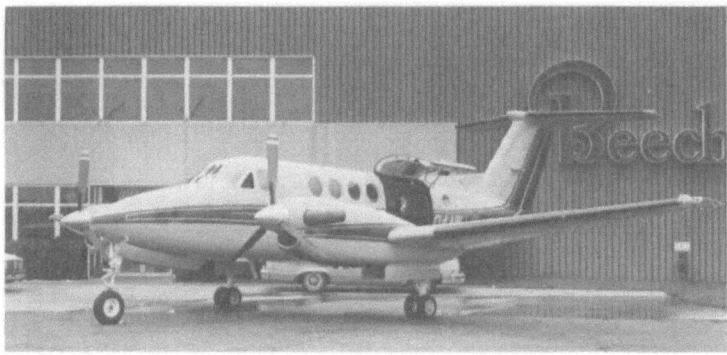

Figure 9. Beech Baron 58. The version shown has the desirable larger cargo door of obvious benefit for the loading of stretchers. (Courtesy of Beech Aircraft Corporation, Wichita, Kansas.)

flown from, and how far it is to the receiving facility. They will also vary according to the climatic conditions to be flown through and whether oceans and mountains have to be crossed.

Adaptability of Aircraft as Air Ambulances

Few if any aircraft have been originally designed with aeromedical care as the primary function. Few if any will be totally suitable as air ambulances, and compromises must be made. A list of presently available aircraft that are adaptable to air ambulance use is provided in Table 1.

The character of the mission must be matched as effectively as possible to the capabilities of the aircraft. Knowledge of the aircraft's primary and secondary characteristics is essential for an informed choice. A checklist for matching the mission to the charter is included in Table 2. Primary and secondary considerations affecting the choice of aircraft are analyzed in the following sections, as are the important characteristics of the mission.

Primary Considerations in Choice of Aircraft

Cabin Space
1. Available floor space
2. Headroom

The amount of care a patient will require during transport will determine the number of medical attendants required and the amount of equipment needed. Comatose patients requiring the continuous use of a respirator and a monitoring system and those on more complex stretchers allowing traction will require more space. Remember that the shape of the curve of the ceiling can severely limit the amount of work room over a stretcher.

Table 1. Aircraft Adaptable as Air Ambulances.

Fixed-Wing	C	MUL	R	S	P	A	RR	E	WL	AC
Cessna Crusader	3	1870	1000	180	No	25(C)	1800	2PE	27.2	230
Cessna 402C	4	1236	1100	180	No	26(S)	2200	2PE	30.3	320
Cessna Chancellor	4	2417	1350	180	Yes 21	30(C)	2600	2PE	29.9	420
Cessna 340	4	2077	1450	180	Yes 20	30(C)	2200	2PE	32.5	320
Beech Baron B55	3	1885	1000	180	No	19(S)	2200	2PE	25.6	180
Beech Baron E55	4	2033	1100	185	No	19(S)	2100	2PE	26.6	220
Beech Baron 58	4	2063	1300	185	No	18(S)	2200	2PE	27.1	260
Beech Baron 58TC	4	2447	1100	185	No	25(C)	2700	2PE	33.0	290
Beech Baron 58P	4	2230	1100	185	Yes 19	25(C)	2700	2PE	33.0	350
Piper Seneca III	3	1898	750	170	No	25(C)	1250	2PE	22.0	200
Piper Aerostar 600A	4	1763	1100	200	No	21(S)		2PE	32.4	260
Piper Aerostar 602P	4	1954	1100	200	Yes 20	25(C)		2PE	33.7	385
Piper Navajo	4	2533	1200	185	No	24(C)	2200	2PE	28.4	375
Piper Navajo CR	4	2441	1300	180	No	24(C)	2300	2PE	28.4	400
Pilatus Britten–Norman Islander	5 (2)	2988	600	150	No	28(S)	1200 UP	2PE	20.3	320
Cessna Titan	6	3616	1500	180	No	26(S)		2PE	34.7	420
Cessna Golden Eagle	5	2860	1200	185	Yes 21	30(C)		2PE	34.7	440
Beech Duke	3	2394	1200	180	Yes 21	30(C)	2700	2PE	31.8	440
Piper Chieftain	4	2824	1300	180	No	24(C)	2500	2PE	30.6	450
Pilatus Britten–Norman Trislander (U.K.)	12 (2)	4250	900	140	No	13(S)	1300 UP	3PE	29.7	480
Cessna Corsair	4	3360	1300	250	Yes 23	30(C)		2TP	36.4	940
Piper Cheyenne	4	3843	1300	240	Yes 25	28(S)	2300	2TP	38.0	970
Piper Cheyenne IIXL	5	4428	1300	250	Yes 25	30(S)	2500	2TP	41.37	1300

Piper Cheyenne III	6	4450	1500	260	Yes 28	32(S)	3200	2TP	37.54	1520
Beech King Air C 90	5	3940	1100	210	Yes 21	28(S)	2300	2TP	41.4	890
De Havilland Twin Otter	7 (2)	5635	750	175	Yes	26(S)		2TP	29.8	NA
GAF Nomad (Australian)	12 (2)	3970	800	175	Yes	23(S)		2TP	20.9	NA
Cessna Conquest	5	4243	2100	300	Yes 28	35(C)		2TP	38.8	1400
Beech King Air B100	5	4793	1400	275	Yes 21	28(S)	2700	2TP	42.2	1400
Beech King Air F90	4	4480	1200	250	Yes 23	29(S)	2900	2TP	39.0	1250
Short Bros Skyvan (U.K.)	10 (4)	5400	950	160	No	22(S)	1500 UP	2TP	33.5	1500
ARAVA (Israeli Aircraft Industries)	10 (4)	66			No		1500 UP	2TP		
Beech Super King Air B200	6	5052	1500	280	Yes 29	35(S)	2900	2TP	41.3	1700
Gulfstream Commander 840	5	3740	2000	275	Yes 23	31(C)		2TP	37.0	1200
Gulfstream Commander 980	5	3642	2000	300	Yes 23	31(C)		2TP	37.0	1500
Gulfstream Commander 1000	5	4040	1500	310	Yes 30	35(S)		2TP	40.0	1600
Embraer Bandeirante (Brazil)	10 (4)	5118	900	235	No	22(S)		2TP	39.9	1500

(continued)

Table 1. Aircraft Adaptable as Air Ambulances (*continued*).

Fixed-Wing	C	MUL	R	S	P	A	RR	E	WL	AC
Pilatus Britten–Norman Turbine Islander (U.K.)	6 (2)	2480	600	180	No	25(S)	1400 UP	2TP	38.2	NA
CASA C 212 Aviocar. (Spain)	10 (4)	6272	950	200	No	28(S)	1500 UP	2TP	38.2	2300
Fairchild–Swearingen Merlin IIIC-23	6	4510	2100	300	Yes 32	31(C)		2TP	45.0	1800
Fairchild–Swearingen										
Merlin IIIC 41	6	5180	2000	310	Yes 32	31(C)		2TP	47.7	1800
Merlin IVC 41	8 (2)	5000	1900	270	Yes 32	31(C)		2TP	45.3	2100
Merlin IVC 41B	8 (2)	5000	1900	270	Yes 32	31(C)		2TP	45.3	2100
Metro III 41	10 (4)	5703	2200	270	Yes 32	31(C)		2TP	45.3	2100
Metro III 41B	10 (4)	5703	2200	280	Yes 32	31(C)		2TP	45.3	2100
Short Bros. 330	24 (6)	7800	750	200	No	19(C)		2TP	49.5	3000
Short Bros. 360 (U.K.)	28 (8)	9200	700	215	No	20(S)		2TP	56.7	3800

Aircraft										
Fokker F-27 (Holland)	40 (8)	17800	1300	250	Yes 20	20(C)	2000	2TP	59.7	6600
de Havilland Dash 7 (Canada)	40 (8)	17056	1200	230	Yes 22	22(S)	UP	4TP	51.2	NA
Lockheed Electra	72 (24)	57000	3000	350	Yes 20	20(S)	4000	4TP	86.9	NA
British Aerospace Intercity 748 (U.K.)	40 (8)	20050	2000	230	Yes 25	25(S)		2TP	56.1	NA
Executive Jets										
Cessna Citation I	6	5395	1500	375	Yes 41	41(C)	3000	2JE	42.5	1700
Citation II	7 (2)	6104	1950	380	Yes 43	43(C)	2400	2JE	41.2	2400
Gates Learjet 25D	6	7150	1600	450	Yes 51	51(C)	4000	2JE	64.7	2300
25G	6	7850	2000	470	Yes 51	51(C)	5000	2JE	71.1	2600
35A	6 (2)	7279	2600	460	Yes 45*	45(C)	4200	2JE	67.2	3300
36A	5	8580	3100	460	Yes 45*	45(C)	5000	2JE	71.1	3400
55	8 (2)	8220	2600	460	Yes 51	51(C)	5000	2JE	73.7	5000
Dassault Falcon 10 (France)	4	7940	2000	450	Yes 45	45(C)	5000	2JE	72.2	4000
20	6	11600	2000	440	Yes 42	42(C)	5250	2JE	65.1	6100
50	8 (2)	18560	3800	450	Yes 45	45(C)	4500	3JE	77.0	9400
British Aerospace HS 125-700 (U.K.)	8 (2)	11300	3000	440	Yes 41	41(C)	5000	2JE	70.3	4700

(continued)

Table 1. Aircraft Adaptable as Air Ambulances (*continued*).

Fixed-Wing	C	MUL	R	S	P	A	RR	E	WL	AC
Rockwell Sabreliner 65	7 (2)	10650	2500	440	Yes 45	45(C)	6000	2JE	63.2	4600
Canadair Challenger (Canada)	8 (2)	21950	3000	440	Yes 45	45(C)		2JE	89.7	8500
Westwind 1	7 (2)	10600	2700	480	Yes 45	45(C)	5000	2JE	74.1	3700
Westwind 2	7 (2)	10900	3200	480	Yes 45	45(C)	5300	2JE	76.2	4400
U.S. Military Airlift Command Aeromedical Evacuation System	[a]									
C-130 Lockheed Hercules	90 (20)	36700	3820	300	Yes	30	4000 UP	4TP		
C-9A Nightingale (McDonnell-Douglas)	40 (10)	35000	1000	450	Yes	25	7000	2JE	107.9	18000
C-141 B Starlifter (Lockheed)	96 (80)	69925	4200	520	Yes	40	6200	4JE	100.0	30000

[a] Carrying capacity numbers as though in civilian use.

Codes for Table 1:

C — Carrying capacity; includes one stretcher patient, does not include cockpit crew. Allowance is made for equipment space. The number below in parentheses represents the number of stretchers that the aircraft can carry on one mission in a manner that each stretcher patient may receive medical attention in flight. Some aircraft can carry many more litters than the number indicated but not in a manner to provide inflight care.

MUL — Maximum useful load (lbs).

R — Range without refueling with 45 minutes to 1 hour reserves. Allowance is also made for adverse weather conditions. Many aircraft can fly farther than the distance indicated with auxiliary fuel tanks. Numbers are statute miles.

S — Speed. This is a mission cruising speed, making allowances for block time—apron waits, taxiing, takeoff, climb to cruising altitude, descent, landing, and parking. It is the speed from which a mission flight time might be estimated if the distance to be flown is known. On longer flights the speed indicated will be too low; on shorter flights it will be too high. Numbers are statute miles per hour.

P — Pressurized, Yes or No. The number shown with Yes represents the altitude at which the cabin can be maintained at 8000 feet. The number followed by * indicates the altitude refers to the cabin maintained at a relative altitude of 6000 feet (numbers in thousands of feet).

A — Altitude ceiling. (S) denotes the service ceiling; (C) denotes this is a certified ceiling above which the aircraft is not permitted to fly. A service ceiling is the highest density altitude at which the aircraft can maintain a 100 feet per minute climb (in thousands of feet).

RR — Runway length required (feet). This not the F.A.R. balanced length rating. The figure allows a mission coordinator to make a preliminary aircraft-airport matching. If the letters UP are shown under the RR number, the aircraft is capable of using unprepared landing strips (nonpaved, grass, dirt).

E — Type of engines (PE, piston engines; TP, turboprop; JE, jet engines).

WL — Wing loading (lbs/sq ft). High-wing-loading aircraft are less disturbed by turbulence.

AC — Approximate cost of a new aircraft in 1982 (in thousands of U.S. dollars).

Manufacturers of aircraft, dealers, brokers, and operators must realize that the numbers quoted are approximations and not necessarily accurate or official figures. They were chosen to indicate to medical flight attendants the capabilities of each aircraft, so that they may ascertain a given aircraft's suitability for the intended uses.

Some older aircraft have been included. They are still in use and have given satisfactory service for the author on aerovac missions.

Table 2.   Checklist for Matching the Mission to the Charter.

Character of the Mission
1. Patient: medical condition and needs in flight (equipment and personnel)
2. Passengers: number of persons who *have* to accompany the patient
3. Dispatching facility: where and what
4. Receiving facility: where and what
5. Distance: between dispatching and receiving facilities
6. Climates: to be left, traversed, and entered
7. Terrain: to be traversed (mountains? oceans?)
8. Urgency: how soon to initiate, how fast to perform
9. Finances available

Character of the Charter
1. Airports or airstrips: length and character of runway and approach; facilities—navigational and servicing (applicable to stopovers and turnaround)
2. Distance: total; between origin and destination; hops between stopovers
3. Payload: patient, attendant(s), equipment, luggage, passengers, flight crew, supplies
4. Terrain and climate
5. Urgency: when available to initiate, dedicated use-time
6. International permits and clearance
7. Primary and secondary characteristics of aircraft
8. Aerovac experience of flight crew
9. Quoted costs

Access Doors
1. Position in fuselage
2. Width
3. Height
4. Height of door bottom above ground
5. Steps and stop wires
6. Method of opening and closing (from inside and out)
7. Relationship of door to C of G (center of gravity)

It should be obvious how 1 through 4 affect the loading and unloading of a patient and determine whether the use of a particular type of stretcher is possible.

Steps are often built into the door and present themselves as the door is opened, hinged at the bottom. How far the door will fall is often controlled by stop wires which attach from the fuselage down to the steps. These stop wires often get in the way when loading a stretcher. When there are two stop wires, one of them can sometimes be detached to make more room for loading the stretcher, remembering that by doing so you reduce the weight the steps are capable of carrying.

Methods of Opening Doors.   Each aircraft seems to have a different arrangement of mechanisms for opening and closing the doors. Unless a medical flight attendant is familiar with the arrangement on the aircraft he is about to use or has been shown how to open and close the doors, it is wise to have the flight crew operate them, as some are easily damaged.

Relationship of the C of G. The relationship of the entrance to the C of G is especially important in light aircraft having a nose wheel. Too much weight behind the C of G can cause the plane to tip tail down. The chances of a tip are greatly ameliorated if the cockpit is occupied and if more than one person *does not* place weight on the steps at one time. Luggage which is going to be stored aft should be loaded last.

Occasionally, when the patient plus accompanying equipment is heavy, it might be necessary for the pilot to run an engine with a propellor giving propulsion with the plane's elevators depressed, giving an upward force to the tail. This gives a counterforce to excessive weight aft of the C of G. This should be avoided if at all possible by being sensible about how weight is distributed on loading and unloading. Should it be necessary in a twin-engined plane, the pilot will use the engine on the side opposite to the entrance, usually the starboard engine. If the plane is at its home base, a tail prop may be available.

Not only is the C of G important on loading and unloading, but the distribution of weight in the longitudinal axis of the cabin can hinder or help the flying ability of the aircraft and affect the safe operation of the plane. How the C of G affects stretcher placement and orientation will be discussed later under Posture, Placement, and Orientation.

Payload

An aircraft can carry a certain payload a certain distance under standard conditions. The weight a medical transport aircraft can carry will have a specific upper limit, which will be reduced relative to the distance the transfer must cover on its longest hop. The heavier the payload, the longer the runway needed. Therefore, if it is known that a runway to be used is of limited length, the payload may need to be reduced.

The payload becomes very important in deciding with the pilot whether one or more persons may be taken on board to accompany the patient. Relatives have a habit of turning up at the airport as a patient is about to be flown out and expected to be able to join the flight. Payload can be used as a tactful excuse should you wish to exclude a would-be passenger from a difficult aeromedical flight.

Range

The range of an aircraft can be increased in a number of ways: by reducing the load, reducing the speed to the optimum cruising speed, and choosing the altitudes and routes most compatible with the capabilities of the aircraft. Wind direction and force have a considerable effect on range, especially with light aircraft which do not have the flexibility of speed or altitude capability of the more powerful planes.

It should be remembered that the range of an aircraft might change during flight due to changes in the weather (even outside temperature can alter range). Therefore, a transfer originally conceived as a single point-to-point flight may change to one requiring a refueling stop, or vice versa. Ranges are usually quoted with a specified flying-time reserve (often 45 minutes).

Speed

The length of time a patient has to spend in flight on a medical transfer is inversely proportional to the cruising speed of the aircraft chosen. Aircraft can fly faster or slower than the recommended cruising speed, but only within limits and at a sacrifice of time or range.

Runway Required

The runway length required by a particular aircraft limits the number of airfields the aircraft can use. A smaller aircraft therefore has certain advantages over a larger one in that it may be able to land nearer to the hospital to which the patient is being transferred, thus reducing the distance a ground ambulance must travel.

When runway lengths are quoted, the height of any obstruction that can be cleared at the end of the runway is mentioned. The payload and whether any reserve fuel tanks are carried may also be mentioned.

Service Ceiling

Knowing the service ceiling of a particular aircraft will give an indication as to whether it is capable of flying at altitudes above turbulent air and thus able to better avoid adverse weather.

Aviation Fuel Used

This would appear to be of more concern to the pilot. Some smaller airfields may not have the particular fuel required for refueling on a stopover or turnaround. This might alter the flight plan for an aeromedical evacuation. It is also a concern for a medical flight attendant in that some fuels present a different degree of danger to the occupants of an aircraft during refueling, both with regard to fumes which might be toxic and increased ignitability increasing the danger of fire (see Refueling).

Secondary Considerations in Choice of Aircraft

Climate Control

Almost all aircraft have some ability to heat or cool the cabin, but with systems having varying degrees of sophistication. It must be remembered that most of the climate control systems are inoperative when the engines are shut down. A refueling stop in a very hot or very cold climate can therefore present problems for the patient. Consideration must be given to removing the patient to more comfortable quarters if the stop will be long enough to adversely affect the climate in the cabin.

Pressurization

Not all aircraft are pressurized. If an aircraft is unpressurized, the maximum altitude at which it may fly without the flight crew using supplementary oxygen is 10,000 feet. A patient may need supplementary oxygen at much lower altitudes and may have conditions adversely affected by the decrease in atmospheric pressure. The effect of low atmospheric pressure on cases of pulmonary and cardiac insufficiency, hypovolemia, and severe anemia will be discussed elsewhere in this book, as will the effect on the airspaces within the body.

Except for the transport of patients with simple musculoskeletal injuries who are in good general health, unpressurized aircraft should not be used for aeromedical flights of any significant distance. However, even when transporting a healthy patient having on a plaster cast for a simple fracture of a limb, certain precautions need to be taken in both pressurized and unpressurized aircraft (see Trauma (extremities)). The pressures to be expected in the cabins of various aircraft flying at different altitudes will be discussed under Oxygenation.

In an emergency, a pressurized aircraft may suddenly lose its cabin pressure. If a plane flying at 31,000 feet has a cabin pressure of 6000 feet and should the cabin become depressurized, the occupants of the cabin would be unlikely to survive for longer than 2 minutes without immediate supplementary oxygen. Emergency oxygen systems were devised to operate automatically at various pressures. The Robertshaw Passenger Oxygen Control system is activated when the cabin altitude exceeds 13,000 feet. When the cabin pressure is restored, the system is automatically turned off as the cabin altitude drops below 12,000 feet.

Many ill or injured patients could not tolerate the pressures to be found at 13,000 feet, or at much lower altitude levels for that matter, without increased oxygenation. Therefore, a medical flight attendant must be able to know the cabin altitude at any time, and an altimeter is essential equipment for his flight bag.

Oxygen Supply

Very few light aircraft have been retrofitted or adapted to provide piped oxygen from a reservoir supply of adequate capacity since such adaptation is very expensive. Without a pipe supply, oxygen cylinders with an adequate capacity and a weight within the imposed restrictions must be carried. Flowmeters and humidifiers that work in the aviation environment must also be available.

Carrying oxygen as compressed gas in cylinders is the most common means of providing oxygen in planes, but other systems are used. These other systems are known as SOX, LOX, and OBOGS. SOX is oxygen produced from a solid state. It is used only as emergency backup supply for short periods. LOX is liquid oxygen. OBOGS is an onboard oxygen-generating system and works by the use of molecular filters. These various systems are discussed in greater detail under Oxygenation.

The connectors of respiratory equipment that might be needed on a flight should be tested to see that they fit the oxygen outlet sockets provided.

Electrical Supply

Some aircraft do have an electrical harness allowing access to outlets providing 110 volts. Others can provide other voltages. The power is generated by the aircraft engines. Some are able to store a limited amount of electrical power in batteries for use when the engines are shut down.

Many aircraft used for aeromedical transfers will not have this luxury, and devices such as monitors and respiratory and suction equipment will require batteries of sufficient capacity to last the length of the flight.

Before any equipment is plugged into an outlet, it must be ascertained whether the outlet provides alternating or direct current and at what voltage. If alternating current, the cycle periodicity must be known.

Electrical equipment carried in aircraft must not generate electrical magnetic interference of a magnitude to interfere with the operation of essential navigational equipment.

Communications Capability
All aircraft used for medical transport will have air traffic control and navigational radio equipment of varying degrees of sophistication. This does not necessarily mean that a medical flight attendant will always have the capability of being in direct radio communication with a medical director or the flight coordinator at home base.

Air to ground radio communications are very important for the efficient air transfer of a patient so that there are minimal delays of the ground transport vehicles meeting the flight and so that the ground vehicle knows where to meet the plane. Medical advice may need to be sought in flight and medical reports given that will be useful for the receiving facility to be better prepared. Air traffic controllers are not able to pass on these messages except in emergencies related to the operation of the aircraft.

Toilet Facilities
Toilet facilities are very limited or nonexistent in most light aircraft. Some of the light jet aircraft and a few of the twin-engined light planes with larger seating capacities do have self-contained sanitary toilets. Privacy is sometimes minimal.

For flights in most light aircraft, urinals and bedpans of the lightest construction will need to be taken on board, with containers for sanitary storage after use.

Refrigeration
Only a few light aircraft have centrally powered refrigerators. The need for a refrigerator is uncommon but occasionally presents itself on longer flights. Alternative methods of cool storage for biological medicines, pathological specimens, and food may need to be used (e.g., small Styrofoam iceboxes).

Rescue and Escape Appliances
Aircraft which are expected to make flights over large tracts of water must carry lifesaving equipment that meets certain standards. An aircraft that has not been operating over water and does not carry this equipment cannot be chartered for a transoceanic medical transfer flight. There must be enough equipment for everyone on board.

Conclusion

The primary and secondary considerations stated above are worthy of note when an air ambulance company is considering the purchase of an aircraft for use in aeromedical work. Other factors that should be considered include the *basic cost of the aircraft, service and maintenance availability and costs,* and whether the particular type and model of the aircraft to be chosen is *still in production* and in what numbers.

FEDERAL AVIATION ADMINISTRATION REGULATIONS: EXCERPTS

The following are some excerpts from the Federal Aviation Regulations which are of some direct and indirect interest to medical flight attendants. They are included here primarily to underscore the importance the authorities place on the safety of flight operations, on the hazards of flying at altitude without supplementary oxygen, and the safety risks related to alcohol and drugs. The regulations on narcotics and other drugs make it imperative that a medical flight attendant be properly licensed in the state in which he practices or resides.

91.70   Aircraft may not operate below 10,000 feet at an airspeed of more than 250 knots unless authorized by the Administrator.

91.32   *Supplemental Oxygen.*
    (a)   General. No person may operate a civil aircraft of U.S. registry—
        (1)   At cabin pressure altitude above 12,500 feet (MSL) up to and including 14,000 feet (MSL), unless the required minimum flight crew is provided with and uses supplemental oxygen for that part of the flight at those altitudes that is of more than 30 minutes duration;
        (2)   At cabin pressure altitudes above 14,000 feet (MSL), unless the required minimum flight crew is provided with and uses supplemental oxygen during the entire flight time at those altitudes; and
        (3)   At cabin pressure altitudes above 15,000 feet (MSL), unless each occupant of the aircraft is provided with supplemental oxygen.

91.11   *Liquor and Drugs.*
    (a)   No person may act as a crewmember of a civil aircraft—
        (1)   Within 8 hours after the consumption of any alcoholic beverage;
        (2)   While under the influence of alcohol; or
        (3)   While using any drug that affects his faculties in any way contrary to safety.
    (b)   Except in an emergency, no pilot of a civil aircraft may allow a person who is obviously under the influence of intoxicating liquors or drugs (except a medical patient under proper care) to be carried in that aircraft.[1]

---

[1] *Author's comment*: As a medical flight attendant, it could be argued that the attendant is a crew member and that 91.11 (a) applies. Regarding (b), this regulation should be considered if a relative or companion wishing to accompany the patient on a flight appears or acts as though intoxicated. Such a person would not be considered to be "a medical patient under proper care" unless a formal arrangement had been made to treat that person as a patient.

91.12   *Carriage of narcotic drugs, marihuana, and depressant or stimulant drugs or substances.*
(a)   Except as provided in paragraph (b) of this section, no person may operate a civil aircraft within the United States with knowledge that narcotic drugs, marihuana, and depressant or stimulant drugs or substances as defined in Federal and State statutes are carried in the aircraft.
(b)   Paragraph (a) of this section does not apply to any carriage of narcotic drugs, marihuana, and depressant or stimulant drugs or substances authorized by or under any Federal or State statute or by any Federal or State agency.

EQUIPMENT AND INVENTORY CONTROL

The Medical Flight Bag

The contents of the medical flight bag should be chosen to offer a limited variety of drugs, medicaments and equipment that will most likely cover the needs of the majority of medical conditions that may require treatment in transit. To accomplish a full and competent preflight assessment of the patient's condition when the necessary diagnostic instruments may not be available at the pickup point, sufficient equipment must be taken in the flight bag.

The choice of contents for the medical flight bag must be influenced by the fact that there are weight and volume restrictions on the equipment that can be carried. This is so because of the payload restrictions of some light aircraft, but also because the medical flight attendant may have to carry the bag a considerable distance.

A proper preflight assessment of the patient's condition made by telephone or radio can indicate what equipment will be essential. The medical flight attendant may find the patient's condition to be quite different from the impression of the condition received prior to arrival. Imagination must be used to predict what might be required beyond that decided upon by preflight assessment. This is especially important in trauma cases.

The amount of equipment to be carried on the outbound leg of the journey can be reduced if, during the preflight assessment, it can be determined what equipment, medications, and fluids will be available at the dispatching facility. When flying to certain parts of the world where supplies are scanty, it may be necessary to determine what needed equipment and medications might be lacking at the reception base or hospital. Arrangements may need to be made to fly in what is necessary.

There are many kinds of medical bags that can be used (Figs. 10–13). Two smaller bags can be used instead of one larger bag. As the majority of medical transfer flights will have only one attendant, a single larger

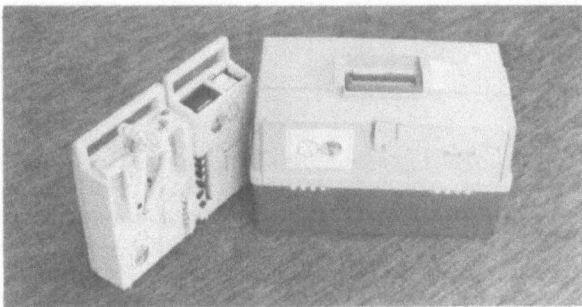

Figure 10.   Flight bag for equipment (Plano 747). Life Pak 5 with defibrillator and monitor.

bag is possibly more useful as it can be carried with one hand and the other hand can be free to carry other equipment. The author's preference is for one flight bag called *Plano 747*, made by the Plano Molding Company and originally designed for holding fishing tackle. The box is made of strong but light plastic, it can carry an incredible amount of equipment, and it is conveniently divided into compartments.

What a flight bag should contain will depend entirely on the nature of the mission to be flown. The maximum amount will be needed for a multiple-trauma victim being evacuated from some underdeveloped country. The inventories presented in Tables 3 and 4 may be too much or too little according to needs, but they can act as checklists to ensure that no essential equipment is omitted.

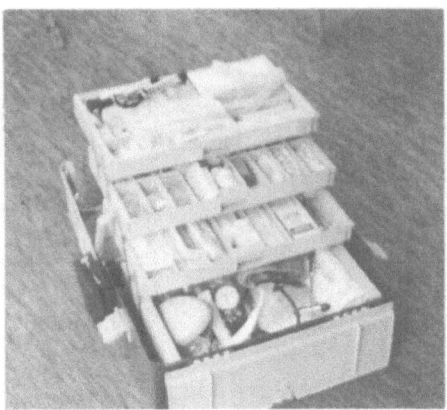

Figure 11.   Plano 747 flight bag showing sliding shelves. Filled with all the equipment for a long distance international mission, the weight may exceed 40 lbs.

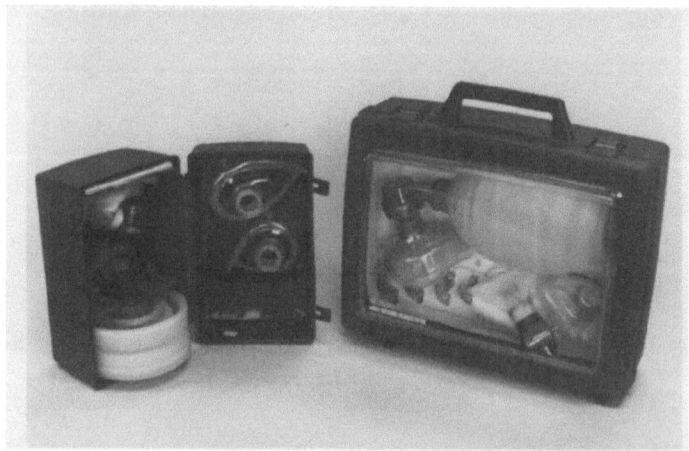

Figure 12.   The Laerdal Company now produces a bag-valve-mask unit using a silicone material for the bag. One advantage is that it can be sterilized by boiling. It is also unaffected by the extremes of temperature likely to be found in the aviation environment. Two types of carrying cases are shown. The bag collapses into itself to be stored in the unit shown on the left. (Courtesy of Laerdal Company, Armonk, New York.)

Inventory

The contents of a flight bag should be checked against an inventory list kept inside the flight bag before each flight, and the condition of the contents and the expiration dates of drugs should be inspected. A copy of the inventory list should be on file at the home base. A record should be kept of what is used, for whom, by whom, and when. Flight bags should be replenished on the completion of a mission and the inventory rechecked.

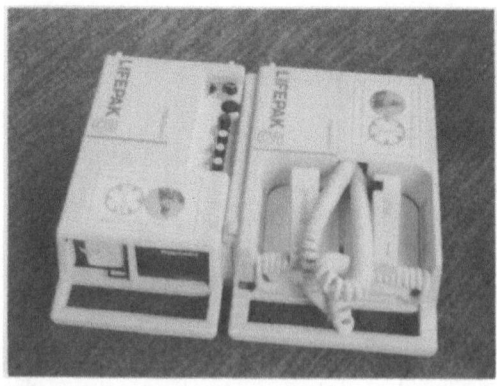

Figure 13.   Life Pak 5. Physiocontrol.

Table 3. Flight Bag Contents—Equipment.

Diagnostic
    Stethoscope
    Ophthalmoscope
    Otoscope
    Laryngoscope (variety of blades)
    Aneroid BP machine
    Penlight
    Neurological hammer (with LT and PP sensory attachments)
Respiratory
    Nasal cannulas and tubing
    Partial rebreathing mask and tubing
    Nonrebreathing mask and tubing
    Venturi mask with adapters
    Laerdal pocket mask with oxygen inlet
    Oropharyngeal airways (3 sizes)
    Nasopharyngeal airways (2 sizes)
    Endotracheal airways (4 sizes)
    Ambu bag
Intravenous
    IV giving sets (2)
    Intracath needles (3 sizes)
    Butterfly needles (3 sizes)
    CVP catheters (2 sizes)
    U-tube connector
    Microfilter
Gastrointestinal
    Gastric tubes (1 small bore, 1 large bore)
Genitourinary
    Foley catheters (2 sizes)
    Urinary drainage bag and tubing
Surgical
    Cut-down/suture set
        Blade handle
        Blades
        Hemostats (2 small-curved)
        Sutures 3 zero plain cagut on needle (2)
                    5 zero monofilament nylon on needle (2)
        Sterile dressings (gauze, Kling, adhesive tape)
Orthopedic
    Cervical collar (Loxley)
    Coban bandages
    Triangular bandages (2)
Syringes
    50 cc, 10 cc, 1 cc tuberculin (1 of each—disposable)
    5 cc (2)
    3 cc (3)
    Assorted hypodermic needles (10)
Miscellaneous
    Peritoneal dialysis catheter
    Chest tubes
    Heimlich valve

(continued)

Table 3.   Flight Bag Contents—Equipment (*continued*).

Equipment that May Be Carried in Separate Containers

Suction
  Battery-powered suction unit
  Suction catheters
Respiratory (see also Fig. 12)
  Ambu bag
  Masks
  Valves
  Extension tubing
  Reservoir bag
Monitor/Defibrillator (see also Fig. 13)
  Physiocontrol Life Pak 5

Special Equipment

Special packs and equipment may need to be carried for:
  The neonate
  The pediatric and obstetric patient
  Those needing orthopedic traction
  The critically ill cardiac patient
  The severely burned patient

Electronic and LED Readout Equipment

There are many pieces of equipment on the market that are supposed to reduce the necessity to digitally feel and count the pulse or manually measure the blood pressure. These pieces of equipment are expensive, require electrical power, are susceptible to inaccuracies, need more attention than they deserve, and detract from the important duty of paying close attention to the patient and his physical condition. They are, therefore, not recommended for use in flight.

Security
While on a mission, the flight bag should accompany the medical flight attendant at all times and never be left unattended in the aircraft or elsewhere. Storage of the flight bag must taken into account its safety from theft and also its safety from damage due to extremes of temperature or humidity.

Narcotics and Controlled Drugs
In the United States, narcotics and controlled drugs will be supplied under the DEA registration number of the physician who is the medical director of the air ambulance unit. Since drugs are often used in other countries and states far from the responsible physician, it is vitally important that they be given maximum security and that accurate records be kept of their use.

It may sometimes be necessary for the medical director to provide a letter explaining the nature of the aeromedical mission and giving references for the appropriate authorities. Such a document can reduce problems that might arise from transporting drugs across boundaries.

The inventory list may need to be presented at security, customs, or immigration points in airports. If the flight bag is to be opened and inspected, the medical flight attendant must always be present and carefully observe the inspection. As soon as possible after the inspection, the important drug items should be rechecked for their presence. The author has lost drugs during an inspection even though he thought he was carefully observing the procedure.

Compatibility of Medical Equipment with the Aviation Environment

Medical equipment that works adequately in a hospital may not perform well when used for aeromedical transfer missions. A number of factors are involved:

1. Stresses of flight: vibration, multidirectional nature of movements in the environment, possible impact, thermal tolerance, barometric pressure reduction (especially sudden decompression).
2. Radiation of excessive electromagnetic interference which can interfere with the electrical and navigational equipment of the aircraft.
3. Endurance: Battery-powered equipment may not have batteries with adequate endurance to provide power for the length of a long flight.
4. Hazardous materials: Materials kept under pressure in cans that are strong enough at sea level may escape if the pressure differential between the cabin pressure and inside the vessel increases. Batteries containing corrosive liquids can be hazardous in flight.

Acceptability of Equipment

There is a large variety of equipment available to treat and monitor patients. There are numerous manufacturers who modify and refine designs and constantly change materials. Some perfectly adequate equipment ceases to be manufactured, and what is still in use may lose access to factory servicing.

Manufacturers do not test all equipment for specific attributes related to its use in flight. It is necessary that this testing take place, as information on the compatibility of equipment is of great importance to those concerned with aeromedical care. Some impartial evaluators test equipment within a framework of how and where the equipment is to be used. However, their conclusions may not necessarily apply to all aeromedical operations.

Should an air ambulance company or medical air evacuation or rescue unit already own equipment that has given some evidence of not functioning well in flight or presenting some hazard, the Foundation for Safety in Medical Instrumentation will test the equipment. The tests would be for the factors of concern and for the safety of those who might operate or use the equipment. Recommendations may be given on how

Table 4. Flight Bag Contents—Drugs and Medicaments.

Amount	Drug	Essential and Useful Drugs[a]	
		Form and Dosage Unit	Proprietary Name
1	Aminophylline	500 mg in 20 ml vial	
2	Atropine	Bristoject 0.1 mg/ml in 10 ml	
1	Bretylium	500 mg in 10 ml	
1	Dexamethasone	4 mg/ml in 5 ml vial	Hexadrol
1	Dextrose	Bristoject 25 g in 50 ml	
2	Diazepam	10 mg in 2 ml amp	Valium
2	Digoxin	0.25 mg/ml in 2 ml amp	Lanoxin
1	Diphenhydramine HCl	25 mg/ml in 10 ml vial	Benadryl
1	Dopamine	200 mg in 5 ml amp	Intropin
1	Edrophonium HCl	10 mg in 1 cc	Tensilon
2	Epinephrine	1 : 1000 1 mg in 1 ml amp	
2	Epinephrine	1 : 10,000 1 mg in 10 ml (Bristoject 1½ inch 22 gauge needle)	
1	Furosemide	100 mg in 10 ml amp	Lasix
1	Hydroxyzine HCl	50 mg in 1 ml, 10 ml vial	Vistaril
1	Isoproterenol	1 mg in 5 ml amp	Isuprel
2	Lidocaine	Bristoject 1% 100 mg in 10 ml	
1	Lidocaine	2 g in 10 ml vial	
5	Meperidine	50 mg/ml in 1 ml Tubex	Demerol, Pethidine

5	Morphine sulfate	10 mg in 1 ml Tubex	
2	Naloxone	0.4 mg in 1 ml amp	Narcan
2	Phenobarbital	65 mg/ml in 1 ml amp	
2	Phenytoin sodium	50 mg/ml in 2 ml amp	Dilantin
2	Prochlorperazine	10 mg in 2 ml amp	Compazine
2	Propranolol	1 mg in 1 ml amp	Inderal
2	Verapamil	5 mg in 2 ml amp	Isoptin, Calan

Medicaments
Afrin nasal spray
Ammonia inhalants
Alcohol swabs
Hydrocortisone cream 1%

Tablets
Aspirin
Tylenol (acetaminophen)
Tylenol with codeine
Mylanta (aluminum hydroxide, magnesium hydroxide, simethicone)
Nitroglycerin (sublingual 1/150 grains)

Bacitracin ointment
Povidone-iodine swabs
Povidone-iodine ointment

Antiemetics
Oral—Meclizine hydrochloride (Bonine, 25 mg chewable)
Dermal—Transderm-V patches

IV Fluids
500 cc 5% dextrose and water
500 cc Ringer's lactate (Hartmann's)
500 cc Haemaccel

[a] Amounts are for a one-patient mission.

Note: Many emergency drug lists contain calcium chloride. The dangers of its use in advanced cardiac care are now recognized. It is purposely omitted from the above list. It might be added should its use as an antidote to propranolol overdose be considered.

Table 5. Acceptable Equipment for Aeromedical Use (Partial List).

Equipment	Date Evaluated
Cardioscopes/Defibrillators/Recorders	
1. Life Pak 3 Portable Battery-operated Defibrillator with Nonfade Cardioscope and Synchronizer, PN 09-00153-0 (operating on internal battery pack)	12/74
2. Physiocontrol Electrocardiograph Recorder PN 09-000143 (only operating on internal battery pack)	12/74
3. Life Pak 4, ECG Monitor, Tapewriter, and Defibrillator PN 09-00264-S/N	10/72
4. Charge Pak PN 09-11415 S/N 0896 (operating on battery pack and 115 VAC 60 Hz)	3/75
5. Life Pak 5 Cardioscope/Recorder Module	12/77
6. Life Pak 5 Defibrillator/Synchronizer Module	5/79
7. Life Pak 5 Battery Pak Charger	
8. Life Pak 5 Nickel Cadmium Battery Pak	
9. Hewlett-Packard Neonatal Monitor, Model 78260A	5/78
(If heart rate module modified to reduce radiated emissions)	8/78
10. Datascope M/D3 Monitor, Defibrillator/Synchronizer	1/80
11. Recorder and Support Module II	
Nebulizer Units	
1. Aquapak Nebulizer 500, with Adapter 921 and Aquatherm Heating Unit 091, S/N 6217	12/74
2. Bird Free-Flow Humidification Kit	71–72
3. Bard-Parker Nebulizer Heater Jacket	10/78, 1/80
Resuscitators	
1. Infant AIRbird Resuscitators	11/75
2. Samson Neonatal Resuscitator (disposable unit)	11/75
3. AMBU Baby Resuscitator with Paedi Valve P/N 13-140-71	4/76
4. Hope II Infant Resuscitator S/N 178-1659-000 (if used with transparent mask and influences of magnetic relief valve are known)	8/76, 2/80
5. Adult Air-Shields AMBU Resuscitator with E-2 Valve and NR Valve	7/78
6. Adult AIRbird Resuscitator with Silicone Bag	7/78
7. Hope II Adult Resuscitator with Midas Mask	7/78
8. Laerdal Adult Resuscitator	7/78
9. Robertshaw Dual Cylinder Portable Resuscitator	10/75
10. Flynn Series III Ventilator with Oxygen-powered Aspirator	8/76, 2/80

Table 5. (*Continued*).

Equipment	Date Evaluated
Resuscitators (*continued*)	
11. Laerdal Child Resuscitator	11/78
12. Laerdal Infant Resuscitator	11/78
Suction Equipment	
1. Gomco Aspirator Portable Pump Model 789 S/ N B47595 (some excessive EMI on test)	10/74
2. Laerdal Suction Unit Failed test on 7/76 due to excessive EMI. Retested 12/81. An off-the-shelf unit again failed, but a unit with a modified motor was tested and was found acceptable. A Laerdal Suction Unit ordered for aeromedical use should specify the modified motor producing less EMI.	
3. SAM Multipurpose Vacuum Pump	3/75
Thermometers	
1. Tempa-Dot Single-use Oral Thermometer	9/76
2. Uni-Temp Single-use Thermometer	9/76
Transport Incubators	
1. Ohio Air-Vac Transport Incubator	6/75
Air Compressors	
(for respiratory therapy devices requiring external source of compressed air)	
1. Ohio High-performance Air Compressor	8/79
2. Aridyne 3500 Medical Air Compressor System	3/80
Closed Urinary Drainage Systems	
1. Dover Urinary Drainage Bag with Flo-Check Valve and with Urine Meter (Will Ross, Inc.)	6/79
2. Dynacor Closed Urinary Drainage Bag	6/79
3. Curity Monoflo Drainage Bag and Curity Urine Meter with Aspirating Port	6/79
Miscellaneous	
1. Frequency Converter—400/60 Hz Model PS-75-426-1 (Unitron, Inc.). Converts 400 Hz three-phase to 60 Hz single-phase power.	12/75
2. Heimlich Valve (Bard-Parker Laboratories). To be placed in line between patient and underwater sealed chest drainage unit.	6/60
3. Litter/Stryker Frame Respirator Mount (Dosco, Inc.). Supports bird MARK 10-14 Respirator on a Stryker Frame. Modified 1978.	12/75
4. Pleur-Evac Adult-Pediatric, Nonmetered Model A-4000 and Pleur-Evac Adult Pediatric, Metered Model A-4010 (Deknatel Div. Howmedica, Inc.). If used with Heimlich Valve.	10/75

Table 6. Equipment Not Acceptable for Aeromedical Use (U.S. Department of Defense).

Cardiac Monitors/Scopes
1. Datascope Cardiotron, Model 650, with Model G Power Module. Unreliable under conditions of aeromedical evacuation. Low quality workmanship and construction.
2. Datascope M/D 2J Monitor/Defibrillator/Synchronizer. Unreliable under conditions of aeromedical evacuation. Scope adversely affected by altitude. Defibrillator adversely affected by vibration.
3. Tektronix 413 Neonatal Monitor and 400 Series Recorder. Susceptible to high levels of radiated interference in 60- and 400-Hz fields. Affected by extreme environmental conditions and vibration.
4. Mennen-Greatbatch Cardio Pak 936S with Recorder. Excessive EMI. Adversely affected by extremes in environmental conditions and vibration.
5. Mennen-Greatbatch Neonatal Monitor Model 744 with Recorder. Excessive EMI. Adversely affected by vibration and humidity.

Blood Pressure Measurement Devices
1. Filac Vital Signs Monitor, Model F-600. Erratic operational characteristics.
2. Infrasonde Electronic Blood Pressure Monitor. Adversely affected by aircraft acoustical noise.
3. Sphygmostat Pulse Monitor, Model P-75. Electrical shock hazard in battery-charging mode (obsolete).
4. Sphygmostat Electronic Blood Pressure Monitor, Model B-300. Erratic operational characteristics (obsolete).
5. Sphygmostat Electronic Blood Pressure Monitor, Model B-350. Adversely affected by aircraft acoustical noise.
6. Somatronix Digital Blood Pressure and Pulse Monitor, Model 307. Adversely affected by aircraft noise and vibration.

Respiratory Monitors
1. Stoelting's Infant Sentry Apnea Alarm, Model 1500 (prior name, AEL). Sensitive to aircraft vibration.
2. Tektronix 413 Neonatal Monitor with 400 Series Recorder. Susceptible to high levels of radiated interference in 60- and 400-Hz fields. Affected by extreme environmental conditions and vibration.

Humidifiers
1. Bennett Cascade Humidifier, Model 1900. Excessive EMI.
2. Bird Immersion Heater. Possible fire hazard (obsolete).
3. Puritan-Bennett Nebulizer with Immersion Heater, Model 126055, PN 12900. Excessive EMI.
4. Bird Heated Nebulizer Tube. Excessive EMI.

Incubators
1. Air-Shields (Isolette) Transport Incubator, Model TI-58. Possible fire hazard. Bassinet flammable. Audible alarm has excessive EMI.
2. Armstrong CARE-ETTE Isolation Incubator, Model 190A. Requires battery pack, securing devices for infant and incubator, vented mattress.
3. Mist-O_2-Gen Transport Incubator, Model TI-700. Excessive EMI. Unacceptable battery pack. CO_2 buildup.
4. Sierracin Cradle Warmer. Excessive EMI. Lack of securing devices (obsolete).

Table 6. (*Continued*).

Ventilators
1. Bennett MA-1 Ventilator. Excessive EMI. Failed during rapid decompression test.
2. Monaghan Volume Ventilator, Model 225. Fluidic components are adversely affected by changes in ambient pressure.
3. Searle VVA Adult Volume Ventilator, Serial No. 7. Excessive EMI—spirometer and humidifier. Equipment malfunctioned at temperature of 40°F, RH 95%.
4. Bird Ventilator Unit, 28 VDC and 110 VAC, 60-Hz Compressors, Battery Pack and Charger (prototypes). Excessive EMI—28 VDC and 110 VAC, 60-Hz Compressors. IMV Bird Respirator tidal volume sensitive to pressure change.
5. Siemens-Elema 900B Servo Ventilator. Excessive EMI. Significant sensitivity to high humidity and varying temperatures. Excessive peak airway pressure during rapid decompression.
6. Bourns BP200 Infant Pressure Ventilator. Excessive EMI. Airway pressure fluctuations during varying temperatures. Excessive peak airway pressure during rapid decompression.

Infusion Systems
1. DIAL-A-FLO Device. Adversely affected by changes in altitude and solution head pressure.
2. Harvard Compact Infusion Pump, Model 975. Deficiency in syringe holders caused syringe walls to deform.
3. IVAC 400, Automatic Self-Regulating IV Infusion Pump. Pumps air. Not configured for convenient transport, securing, handling, and withstanding vibration (obsolete).
4. IVAC Model 500, Automatic Self-Regulating IV Infusion Pump. Excessive EMI. Adversely affected by changes in cabin pressure (obsolete).
5. Sigmamotor TM-20-2 Infusion Pump. Excessive EMI.
6. Sigmamotor VOLUMET Infusion Pump. Excessive EMI when operating from 115 VAC, 60–400 Hz power.

Suction Units
1. Laerdal Suction Unit. Excessive EMI. Motor overheats. Collection bottle too small.[a]
2. IMPACT Vacuum Pump. Excessive EMI. Unacceptable plug. Electrical shock hazard.

Cast Cutters
1. Stryker Cast Cutter Plaster VAC, Model 845. Exceeds EMI limits. Operates only from 115 VAC, 60 Hz.

Oxygen Equipment
1. Blount Oxygen Flow Meter. Incorrect flows.

Closed Urinary Drainage Systems
1. Abbott Drainbag 2000. Excessive positive pressure in system during rapid decompression.
2. Travenol Cystoflo II Urinary Drainage Bag. Excessive positive pressure in system during rapid decompression.

[a] This applies to off-the-shelf models. Note the comments on the model in the "acceptable" list.

equipment can be modified to make it compatible with the environment in which it is to be used and to make it safe. The Foundation charges modest fees for testing equipment. The fees amount to a contribution to the Foundation, which also provides speakers on safety in medical instrumentation.[1]

An excellent source of information is the Aeromedical Systems Branch of the U.S.A.F. School of Aerospace Medicine (SAM) located at Brooks Air Force Base, Texas 78235. SAM issues reports on medical items tested and evaluated for use in the U.S.A.F. aeromedical evacuation system. Items tested are classified as acceptable equipment, acceptable equipment no longer manufactured, and unacceptable equipment. The reports point out that the acceptability/nonacceptability designations apply only to the routine use of the particular item in the unique aeromedical evacuation environment of the Department of Defense and are not intended as representations to be relied upon by persons or entities outside of the Department of Defense.

The testing done by SAM is extensive, and the reports give indications of why various items are considered unacceptable and how modifications might make them acceptable. It is likely that the reports have influenced manufacturers to make modifications which have enhanced the safety and usefulness of many items.

The SAM lists of acceptable equipment (as of March 1981) are provided without comments or details of the reports (Table 5). Some of the items on the acceptable list have reports which indicate possible hazards if used inappropriately or under certain conditions. The provided unacceptable list is abbreviated but gives some reasons as to why the item was not acceptable at the testing (Table 6). The Aeromedical Systems Branch of SAM is anxious that its evaluations be available in the interest of air evacuation safety.

DOCUMENTATION

With the exception of a helicopter transferring a patient directly from one hospital to another or performing a rescue pickup and flying directly to a receiving facility, aeromedical transfers involve more "steps" than the usual transfer by ground ambulance. There are, in fact, multiple transfers.

1. Dispatching hospital (or site of pickup): ground ambulance
2. Takeoff field: Flight (may be divided into hops involving stopovers requiring ground ambulances)
3. Landing field: ground ambulance
4. Receiving hospital (or site of delivery)

---

[1] Inquiries should be addressed to: Irwin M. Kane, BS, CCE, (Director), Foundation for Safety in Medical Instrumentation, 240 Coachlight Square, Montrose, New York 10548.

It can be imagined that a considerable amount of coordination is required to ensure a smooth transfer at each step. This coordination is primarily the responsibility of a *flight mission coordinator* who should be in close consultation with a medical director or the chosen medical flight attendant.

Medical records may need to be transferred at each stage in order that those accepting responsibility for the care of the patient (be it only for a short time) are aware of the patient's condition and needs.

A medical flight attendant will not always supervise all stages of a transfer. The ideal situation of benefit to the patient is when the medical flight attendant accepts responsibility at the dispatching hospital and remains with the patient until he hands over responsibility to those at the receiving facility. This can usually be done on flights within one country, but on international transfers it is not always possible for the flight attendants to leave the aircraft or the airport.

When the first leg of a transfer using a ground ambulance is long, much time could be wasted by having the flight attendant travel to the dispatching facility. Political situations and national policies may also prevent a flight attendant from leaving a foreign airport to fetch the patient.

With multiple transfers of responsibility, it is important that medical records are accurate, clear, and complete to the extent of their usefulness for the patient's benefit. Sometimes, however, record-keeping is overdone. I have seen a medical flight attendant write voluminous notes during a mission with multiple seriously injured patients while one patient was in urgent need of adjustment of the airway. There are right and wrong times to be writing medical records.

All medical records have some degree of relevancy, even when describing a negative finding. It is the degree of relevancy that should influence what information is worth recording. This might sound strange to physicians and nurses not practicing in the U.S. In the U.S. there is a tendency to document the relevant and the irrelevant. This has created an expensive monster of doubtful use. Standard forms can simplify record-keeping as long as it is realized that the extent to which they are completed should be flexible, and the form should not limit the entry of additional information if it is important.

Service Record

The coordination of the mission demands a record documenting the identity of the individuals concerned:

1. Hospitals
2. Companies providing transport vehicles (ground and air)
3. Interested organizations (employing corporation, consulate) (Fig. 14)

The record should show how each can be contacted, where, and when.

Flow Sheet

When multiple communications are being made during the coordination of a mission, it is useful to use a flow sheet to check off which communi-

Aeromedical Transfer Service Form		
Date: Patient: Age: Sex:		
Time: Home address: Wt:		
Home tel #:		
Who or What	**Address**	**Tel #.**
Patient's private MD		
Hospital (on site)		
Physician (on site)		
Receiving hospital		
Hospital MD contact		
Air Ambulance Co.		
Mission Med. Dir.		
Mission coordinator		
Air Charter Co.		
Charter contact		
Corporation		
Corporate Rep.		
Corporate Med. Dir.		

Medical Problems

Illnesses: Injuries: Date

Med. investigations: Lab:

                       X-rays:

Treatment: Surgery: Date

Can patient walk?   Sit?   Speak English?   Urinary Cath.?

Casts?   Traction?   Splints?   I.V.s?

Monitored?   Intubated?   Ventilator?   Gastric tube?

Equipment needed
on mission?

Time here?   Local (on site) time?

Here: Airport: Runway length: Amb. service:

There:

Who is requesting transfer?   Form completed by:

Figure 14.   Documentation. Aeromedical transfer service form. (Courtesy of International Medical Network, Alexandria, Virginia.)

cations have been made, noting the time of contact or completion (Fig. 15).

Preflight Evaluation Record

Preflight Assessment

Preflight evaluation of the patient who may require transfer by air is vitally important in order that proper medical decisions be made as to the feasibility of transfer (Fig. 16). The preflight assessment also determines the level of service the patient will require, what sort of medical escort will be necessary, what equipment and drugs must be carried, and what type of aircraft will be suitable.

Most preflight assessments will be made from a distance by telephone or radio. Warnings must be given regarding distant evaluation. Experience has shown that preflight assessments made over long distances, especially to other countries by telecommunications, can sometimes be misleading and not have a high degree of validity. There are a number of reasons for this:

1. Quality of telecommunications
2. Language problems
3. Inaccurate information relayed

Telephone communications are presently quite good to most parts of the world when the direct dialing system is used. All preflight evaluations will not be conducted by this system, and it must be expected that some will have to be conducted with transmissions of poor quality. The length of time available to make the communication may also be limited.

Conversations with medical personnel in other countries can be difficult and cause the collection of inaccurate information due to language or dialect differences, or to differences in terminology. Other inaccuracies in communications might be related to the level of competence of those providing the information, or those providing the information see no relevancy in what might be important to the one seeking the information.

Unfortunately, there can be another reason for inaccurate information. Information can be given that is purposely biased to encourage either transfer or nontransfer. A hospital or country may be eager to have a patient transferred out of its jurisdiction earlier than the condition of the patient should allow. Occasionally, a physician or surgeon will not encourage transfer because he wants to maintain responsibility for the care of the patient longer than the patient desires. His medical report could be biased in the direction of the postponement of the transfer. Although these circumstances are unusual, their possibility should be kept in mind when making a preflight assessment from a distance.

Bedside Evaluation

A medical flight attendant must sometimes alter his judgments formed as the result of distant evaluation upon closeup examination of the patient. A thorough bedside evaluation is necessary to confirm information received before the flight. During this bedside assessment, neck fractures or dislocations and intrathoracic or pelvic injuries may come to light.

Special precautions should be taken when evaluating patients with ocular injuries, hemothorax, pneumothorax, head injuries, and intestinal

Aeromedical Transfer: Service Flow Record			
Date:	Time:	Patient:	Sign
		Service call received	
		Med. Dir. informed	
		Responsible party called	
		On site MD called	
		On site hospital called	
		On site ambulance called	
		Private MD called	
		Receiving hospital called	
		Mission coordinator called	
		Flight company called	
		Pilot called	
		Med. flight attendant(s) called	
		Receiving ambulance called	
		Preflight assessment (distant) made	
		Equipment ready	
		(Over and above) medications ready	
		Flight bag checked	
		International documents (personnel)	
		International documents (aircraft)	
		Airline reservations called	
		Airline Med. Dir. called	
		On site hotel called	
		Cash arranged	
		Other	

Information:

Figure 15. Documentation. Aeromedical transfer service flow record. (Courtesy of International Medical Network, Alexandria, Virginia.)

Preflight assessment				
Distant evaluation	Info received from:-		Date/Time:	
Bedside evaluation	Hospital:-			

Patient:-	Age:	Sex:	Wt:	Ht:

Diagnoses   **Date of Onset**
1.
2.
3.
Diabetes?   Insulin?   Allergies?   Ear/sinus problems?
General Condition
Px.

Mental Attitude   **Hgb/Ht.**

Surgery	**RS** O_2 mask type? Flow:
	Type of airway?
	Type of ventilator? Setting:
	Suction required?
When?	Last ABG (R.A. or O_2 flow)

Current Meds	**CVS**
	Has there been arrhythmia? Type:
	How was it treated?
Meds contraindicated.	Reading of last EKG
	CHF? Now? When: How treated.
Meds needed in transit.	Present BP and pulse
	GU Continent? Catheter?
	Adequate kidney function?
Equipment needed/transit.	**Skeletal**
	Traction? Type? Wts.
	Casts? Special stretcher?

	CNS LOC?
Any Med problems of	Present level OC
those accompanying?	Eye signs
	Paralysis?
	GI Eat? Drink? NG tube?
	Colostomy? Last BM:

Receiving Hospital: Name of contact: Date/Time
Has bed been assigned?   Bed #   To whom should you report?
Distance from airport?   Ground ambulance arranged?
                    Ambulance Co. name: Tel:
What accommodations available, near hospital or airport, for flight
and Med crew?
Hotel tel:_____   Signed:_____
Remarks: Printed name:

Figure 16. Preflight assessment form. (Courtesy of International Medical Network, Alexandria, Virginia.)

obstruction because of the adverse effect of the aviation environment without compensatory care.

A further difficulty in making distant preflight evaluations by communication with medical personnel in countries other than the United States is that the propensity for voluminous written medical records often does not exist. It is not that uncommon in some foreign hospitals, even where sophisticated medical services are present, for the records of a patient who has been hospitalized for many days to accumulate only a few pages of notes of a brief nature. Information is often stored in the heads of physicians and nurses and frequently in a log book kept by the Sister or head nurse of a ward. It may be necessary to talk to the doctor *and* the nurse in charge in order to obtain sufficient information.

Unfortunately, the excess of information that might be available from hospital records of a patient in the U.S. can be a hindrance to a clear preflight assessment from a distance. Voluminous records do not guarantee that a clear and accurate assessment can be communicated.

The example of a preflight assessment form (Fig. 16) should not need to be completed in full for every patient. The basic medical conditions prompting the patient's transfer must guide the assessor to the extent of information necessary for a safe medical transfer.

Mission Report

A mission report is a record of the important medical details pertaining to the care of the patient in flight and his condition on transferal to someone else's responsibility (Fig. 17). It should also contain information of a nonmedical nature such as what aircraft was used, the points between which the transfer was being made, and the names of the flight crew. Medications that are given should also certainly appear on the mission report.

Drug-Use Form

At the end of a flight, a drug-use form (which should be carried in the medical flight bag) should be completed so that an inventory of medications is always available and the flight bag is not depleted of essential medications when the next mission is flown (Fig. 18).

Aircraft Documentation

All aircraft must carry documents relating to the operation and airworthiness of the aircraft. A log of the flight is also kept, as is a copy of the flight plan (manifest).

When international borders are crossed, other documents are necessary covering entry and exit formalities, health regulations, customs, and excise. These are the responsibility of the pilot in command, but they become of interest to the medical flight attendant should the attendant disembark at a foreign airport. A list of medical equipment, drugs, and medications that might enter the country with the attendant must be available for the authorities at the airport in order to prevent undue delays in receiving clearance for their entry and exit.

Mission Report	Patient:					Age: Wt:
Date:	From:			To:		
Diagnosis: 1.		2.			3.	

Log	Date Time	Date Time	Cabin altitude	V/S	Intake/ output	Progress notes Meds. O_2 LOC monitor
Pickup						
Arr. airport						
Take-off						
Level-off						
Land						
Disembark						
Arr. Rec. Facility						
Stops						
Land						
Take-off						
Land						
Take-off						
Expenses	$ ¢					
Equipment/ supplies						

Med. Dir: Med. Fl. attendant(s):

Flight crew: Ambulance (pickup):

Aircraft: Ambulance (Rec.):

Comments:

Figure 17. Mission report form. (Courtesy of International Medical Network, Alexandria, Virginia.)

Drug Use Form				
Flight bag no.:	**Premission Inventory Check**			
	Date:		Time:	
	By:			
Mission. Date:	From:		To:	
Patient:				

Date: Time:	Medication	Amount	Given to:	By:

Figure 18. Drug use form. (Courtesy of International Medical Network, Alexandria, Virginia.)

Documentation of Consent and Release

Medical transport by air has definite advantages over ground transport with regard to speed and comfort, when appreciable distances are involved, or when the terrain is difficult to traverse by ground ambulance.

In general, flying is just as safe, or safer, than being transported by ground ambulance. However, some injuries and medical conditions are more susceptible to alterations experienced in the aviation environment, foreseen or unforeseen. The type of aircraft chosen for medical transport, the equipment used, and the employment of qualified flight and medical crew to perform a mission can all contribute to the safety and comfort of the patient. When every precaution has been taken to care for the patient's well-being, something may happen that can aggravate an illness or injury.

Consent and Release Form (81MC 7)

The medical representatives of **MediCall International** have determined, from the information available to them, that:

The patient_____should be able to be transported by air with a medical escort from_____to _____, utilizing ground ambulance for that part of the journey for which it is necessary. However, the aviation environment has variable elements which, at times, can present some risks to the physical condition of the patient, especially when a medical condition or injury already exists.

I,_____(Patient)/_____
(Responsible Party) understand the above and agree to release **MediCall International** from responsibility for any aggravation of illness or injury incurred during transport, and hereby give consent to transport the patient by air.

Signed_____Date_____
Witness_____

The medical representatives of **MediCall International** have determined, from the information available to them, that:

The patient_____has medical conditions which contra-indicate the transfer of the patient by air ambulance. The opinion has been provided that transport by air or ground ambulance may aggravate the illness or injury.

I,_____(Patient)/_____
(Responsible Party) understand the above risk and have made the decision that such a risk should be taken in order that the patient may be transferred from_____to_____and release **MediCall International** from any responsibility for any aggravation of illness or injury, and hereby consent to the transport of the patient by air.

Signed_____Date_____
Witness_____

Note: When it is judged that the risks of transport are such that there is a likelihood that aggravation of illness can occur, **MediCall International** reserves the right to refuse to transfer the patient.

Figure 19. Consent and release form. (Courtesy of International Medical Network, Alexandria, Virginia.)

In the atmosphere of litigation that exists in the United States, certain documents on which signed consent can be demonstrated are useful. Signed forms can document that the patient and/or those responsible for him had knowledge of the risks involved and were given the opportunity to take part in the decision to face those risks (Fig. 19).

There are two situations to be covered by consent and release forms when transporting a patient by air:

1. There are no obvious contraindications to transporting the patient by air in a properly equipped aircraft, and the transfer is in the medical interest of the patient or at the patient's request for his own convenience.

2. The air ambulance company and its medical director provide the opinion that the medical transfer by air is contraindicated according to the seriousness of the patient's illness or injuries, but agree to transport the patient with due consideration of the risks involved.

This would not commonly happen, but there will be situations where the risks of an aeromedical transfer must be balanced against those risks of leaving the patient in the circumstances in which he finds himself. An air ambulance company should always have the right to refuse to transfer a patient when the transfer by air is medically contraindicated.

LOADING AND UNLOADING

During aeromedical transfers, most untoward incidents occur during loading or unloading of the patient.

Stretchers

When a patient is seriously ill or injured, each transfer from one supporting structure to another is an inconvenience, a discomfort, or an added chance for trauma. A scoop-breakaway stretcher can reduce the number of poorly supported patient moves from one structure (bed or other stretcher) to another (Fig. 20).

The location and size of the entrance of most light aircraft necessitate using a stretcher of modest width and one which has an adjustable length. The weight of the stretcher should offer a minimal burden to the personnel who will have to lift it and to the payload of the aircraft. The adjustable scoop-breakaway stretcher is the most suitable to fit these requirements.

The patient must be well-secured when using the scoop stretcher, because loading and unloading sometimes necessitates lifting the stretcher at a relatively steep angle to the horizontal. Upper-thigh straps similar to those used on long spine boards may need to be applied.

A patient may be "scooped" from the bed at the origin of the transfer and remain on the scoop until "unscooped" onto the bed in the receiving

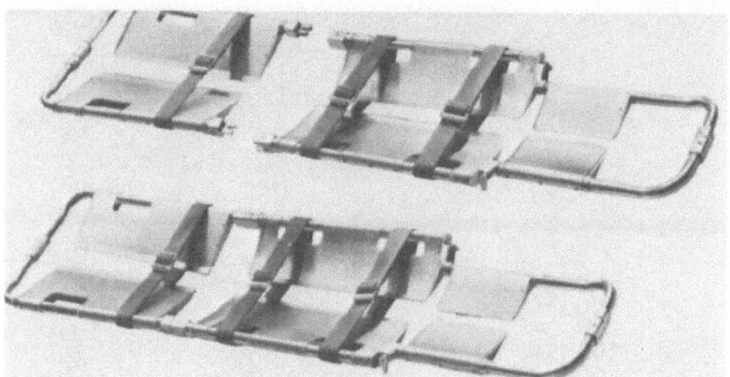

Figure 20.   Ferno-Washington Model 69-X orthopedic scoop stretcher. The foot section is extendable. If the scoop is removed from the patient in the aircraft, it can be taken apart and stored without creating a space problem. (Courtesy of Ferno-Washington, Inc., Wilmington, Ohio.)

facility. This may mean the patient could be on the scoop for many hours. Some scoop stretchers are made with leather-like material as the sling support. The tension of the sling can be released, allowing the patient to be supported by the mattress of the stretcher on which the scoop rests. Other scoop stretchers are all-metal. They can be temporarily broken open to give the patient more comfort for a longer period of time or removed altogether if it is certain a similar scoop is available to unload the patient.

Advantages of Scoops
Most scoops are light in weight. They can be placed under the patient without moving him too much, their length can usually be adjusted, and extra length can sometimes be used for the attachment of traction devices. They are also not as wide as other types of stretchers.

Disadvantages of Scoops
A patient secured to a scoop cannot be postured in a sitting or semisitting position. As far as the author knows, no scoop has been manufactured entirely out of a material other than metals, which present a conductive hazard in monitoring and electrical defibrillation. (Insulated, padded covers for the blades of a scoop stretcher or its manufacture in a light, nonconductive material would be welcome.)

The Vacuum Mattress
Not many of this type of stretcher are used in the United States, but they are commonly used in Europe. Deutsche Rettungsflugwacht (German Air Rescue) and S.A.M.U. (Service Aide Medical d'Urgence) of Paris use a version of the vacuum stretcher (Fig. 21).

The stretcher consists of a mattress containing a myriad of plastic beads. In its softened state, it can be molded around the patient in any

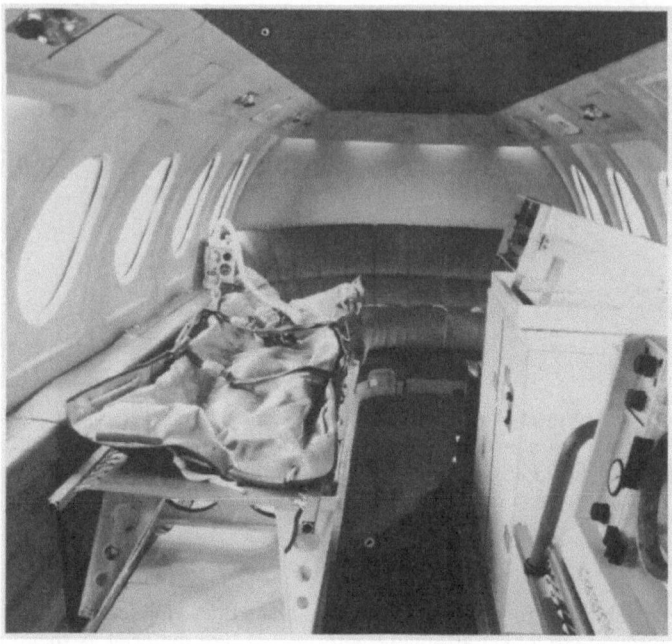

Figure 21. Vacuum stretcher shown in a Falcon 50. (Courtesy of Dassault International, Vaucresson, France.)

shape to give support and comfort. After air is withdrawn from the mattress by means of a hand-operated air-suction pump, it becomes rigid and maintains its configuration until air is reintroduced.

Vacuum stretchers are somewhat bulky, and securing a patient to one with straps is more difficult than with a rigid scoop. They do have the advantage of being nonconductive and radiotranslucent. They are possibly of greatest use for multiple fractures, especially those of the thoracic and lumbar spine, pelvis, and lower limbs. They do have rope- or strap-carrying handles, but they are not as easily handled when they have to be lifted at an angle to load a patient into an aircraft.

Loading

Before the mechanics of the actual lifting and manipulation of the stretcher are discussed, points regarding the preparation for loading need to be addressed (Fig. 22).

1. The ground ambulance should be as near to the aircraft entrance as is convenient, making allowances for the safety of the aircraft. Its position should be taken with the guidance of the pilot.

2. Before the doors of the ground ambulance are opened, the cabin of

the aircraft should be checked to make sure that any movable hindrances to loading are moved out of the way. The aircraft stretcher which will support the one on which the patient is being loaded should be checked to see that it is properly secured to the floor and that the oxygen cylinders are rigidly secured.

The oxygen cylinders should be cracked and ready to connect if needed. If possible, the climate in the cabin should be made hospitable. Note should be made of where any IV reservoirs will be attached, so that there is minimal delay in checking the adequacy of the IV flow.

3. A minimum of three persons are required for loading. All those who will be assisting with the loading should be briefed on the plan of loading. If the pilot is experienced in aeromedical transfers in the particular aircraft being used, he should direct the loading; otherwise, the medical flight attendant should direct the loading, noting any advice from the pilot regarding the structure of the entrance steps, the influence of the center of gravity of the aircraft, and the parts of the aircraft that must not bear weight.

4. Before the patient is lifted from the ground ambulance, any oxygen tubing, IV lines, or drainage tubes should be adjusted to limit the possibility that they will be caught on some projection during the loading process. *If there is a loop that might be caught, it will be caught* is a maxim to be remembered.

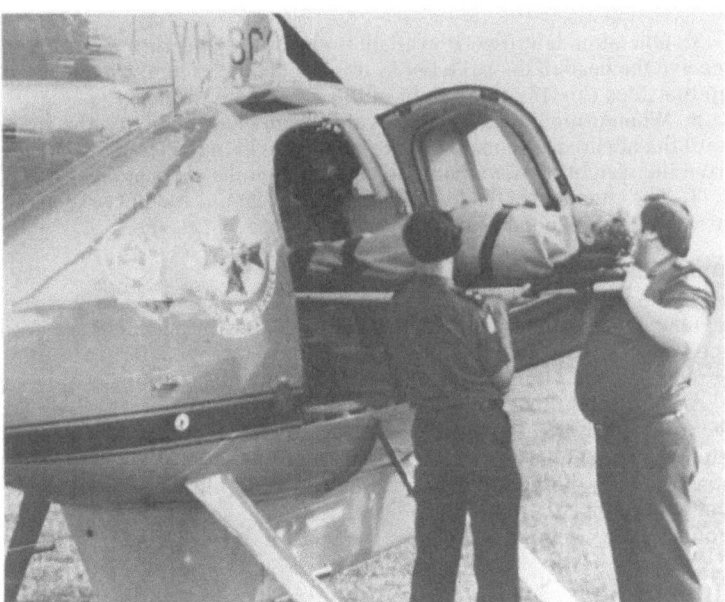

Figure 22.   Loading a patient into a 500D helicopter. Note the height to which the stretcher must be lifted. (Courtesy of Hughes Helicopter, Inc., Culver City, California.)

Pliable intravenous fluid reservoirs can be placed under the patient's shoulder or arm to maintain flow during loading. Glass IV bottles should be avoided whenever possible; but should one be in use, it is probably wise to temporarily close the flow during the loading and to secure the bottle to the stretcher near the head with adhesive tape to reduce the chance of breakage.

5. If the medical flight attendant has not accompanied the patient on the journey to the plane, he should be briefed on any change in condition of the patient during that journey. Medical records from the dispatching hospital should be transferred.

Hints on Loading

Although it has been mentioned that a minimum of three persons is required to load a patient, five or six is not too many. Two persons of normal strength can easily carry one patient on a scoop stretcher if the patient is of moderate weight and there is no oxygen cylinder between his legs (that is, if the stretcher is carried horizontally at a level so that the carriers' arms are hanging in full extension).

To lift the same stretcher and its load up to shoulder height is difficult; to do this with the stretcher at various angles, with longitudinal rotation being carefully controlled, is even more difficult. Those who have never had the experience of loading a patient into a light aircraft or up a ground step ramp into a large aircraft should practice lifting a loaded scoop stretcher up to someone standing on a large table in order to appreciate the effort involved.

1. One attendant (two if available) should be aboard the aircraft to receive the head of the stretcher as it is handed up to him. Do not climb up the steps carrying the weight of the head of the stretcher.

2. When using a light aircraft, avoid placing any weight on the steps until the attendant on board has the main weight of the stretcher. Never have the weight of more than one attendant on the steps at one time.

3. The attendant at the foot of the stretcher should attempt to keep the stretcher as horizontal as is practical and to prevent rotation.

Immediately after Loading

Once the patient is on board, attend to the oxygenation equipment and regulate the flow if it is immediately required. Secure and adjust the IV if one is needed. Should the IV have infiltrated or stopped during loading or during ground transport, restart it *before* the plane begins taxiing.

All equipment that might be needed should be made accessible and secured. Secure the patient to the stretcher and the stretcher supports. After the patient has been attended to, notify the pilot that relatives (or others joining the flight) may embark. The pilot will direct the seating and securing of the other passengers. Luggage should be loaded and stowed at the appropriate time by the cockpit crew.

Unloading

Much time can be saved by thinking ahead, and preparations for unloading should commence during the descent of the aircraft well before the final approach. Once the final approach has commenced, the attendant will be seated and belted and will not have the opportunity to move about the cabin freely.

The descent of the aircraft has more effect on the patient physiologically than did the ascent, so the attendant must be prepared to closely attend to the patient and be ready to deal with any vomiting that may occur and advise on amelioration of barometric effects on the ears and sinuses. For this reason, preparations for unloading need to be started very early on during the descent.

Preparations include completing the charting of medical records so that there will be minimal delay in transferring records to those receiving the patient on landing. Hindrances to unloading should be moved, and further movement prevented by securing. Confirmation by radio that the ground ambulance crew will be waiting and are aware of the E.T.A. and the location within the airport where the meeting will take place should be completed.

The same precautions that were recommended for loading now apply just as rigidly for unloading, and each unloading should be preplanned with the resources available, again remembering that: *During aeromedical transfers, most untoward incidents occur during loading and unloading.*

ORIENTATION AND POSTURE

Orientation of the Stretcher in Aircraft

There is still considerable controversy regarding the direction in which the patient's head should be placed during medical transport by air. Some authorities have continued the opinion that patients with cardiac problems should be transported with the head toward the rear of the aircraft, and those with cerebral edema, the reverse. This opinion is based on the effect of acceleration and rate and angle of climb of the aircraft on the physiology of the patient.

The problem is not as simple as that. It is suspected that the above opinion was formed before aircraft acquired the ability to brake effectively in order to shorten the necessary runway length required to land the larger planes and fast, light aircraft. Nowadays, the forces of deceleration are almost equivalent to those of acceleration.

If the first opinion is to influence us as to how we orientate the patient, we may have to turn the patient around at the midpoint of the flight. This is hardly possible in a light aircraft whose cabin width is less than the length of a stretcher.

Factors to be Considered

Tradition.   Tradition can interfere with reasonable thought in some circumstances. Traditionally, when a patient is moved in a horizontal attitude, he is moved longitudinally. This has been a reasonable tradition for wheeling stretchers along corridors and for loading into ambulances.

The compartments of ground ambulances are longer than they are wide, and the width is usually not sufficient to allow for sideways orientation of the stretcher. Even if the compartments did allow sideways transportation of the stretcher, the forces present as the vehicle turned corners would be more annoying than with the stretcher fore and aft. The fore and aft forces of acceleration and deceleration can be minimized by thoughtful driving. These facts have reduced the necessity to consider transporting patients in other than the longitudinal axis of the vehicle's compartment. This tradition of fore and aft orientation has persisted and transferred its influences, to some degree, to air ambulances.

Cross-Plane Orientation.   Placing the stretcher across the cabin instead of fore and aft has some advantages. The forces of acceleration and deceleration can cause considerable shift of body fluids. If these forces are acting on the longitudinal axis of the body, the blood flow to the cranial contents can be decreased or excessive depending on the direction of the forces in relationship to the patient. The cardiovascular system can be insulted by the movement of body fluids, with increase or decrease in cardiac input and loss of fluid to the circulating volume. When the patient is at right angles to these detrimental forces, these forces are of much less importance to the vital functioning of the body. The detrimental effects of longitudinal forces have been demonstrated by experiments on anesthetized animals in which sagittal sinus pressures increased up to 30% on maximum power takeoffs with the animal transported with headaft.

Lateral forces on cornering of ground vehicles have been mentioned. When an aircraft makes a standard turn (the correct banking angle for the speed and rate of turn), it converts much of the centrifugal force to one acting downward in relationship to the floor of the aircraft. This ameliorates shifts of body fluids that might occur in the head-foot direction in a patient transported in a cross-plane orientation. In this respect, the skill of the pilot can benefit the patient.

Dominant Attitude of Aircraft.   The dominant attitude of fixed-wing aircraft is nose-up on climbing and landing. A plane does not always follow its nose on a downward angle except when diving. On normal descents, the aircraft sinks, maintaining an almost horizontal attitude. The final glide just before landing is usually in the nose-up attitude until the main landing wheels have caught and the nose wheel has landed. In the case of aircraft with tail wheels, the nose up attitude is maintained after landing and is actually increased as the tail wheel is allowed to take weight.

It is usually not comfortable or desirable for one's head to be lower than one's feet for any length of time. There are only a few times when it would be indicated medically. This information would suggest that a patient would be more comfortable with the head forward if he must be transported longitudinally to the fore and aft axis of the cabin. If there are overriding reasons why the head should be aft, it is conceivable that the stretcher could be angled so that the head is not lower than the feet when the plane is nose-up.

Center of Gravity.   If a patient is placed in a light aircraft with the head facing aft, depending on the placement of the stretcher in the cabin, the aircraft may be well-balanced. However, should the patient require intensive care such as endotracheal intubation, or should respiratory or other equipment need to be moved aft and the medical flight attendant moves behind the patient, balance may be compromised.

There is, of course, some alteration of balance when extra weight moves forward, should the patient's head he toward the front. The "unloaded" center of gravity is more forward than aft within the available cabin space, so there is less effect on the flying ability of the aircraft than when extra weight is moved aft.

Do not get the impression that there is such a delicate balance that the plane will become unsafe with any shifts in weight distribution. The point is that sensible weight distribution within the part of the cabin to be used by the medical flight attendant is beneficial to the easy control of the aircraft and to the comfort of the patient. This should be recognized by the medical flight attendant when he cooperates with the pilot in deciding where to place the stretcher.

Other Passengers on Board.   When passengers, such as relatives and friends, are accompanying the patient, it is preferable that they be seated aft. This way the medical flight attendant, with the patient, can be closer to the flight deck and can communicate closely with the flight crew. In the event that procedures may need to be performed on the patient that would be upsetting to the other passengers, some sort of screening may be possible to separate the passengers from the "action." These considerations also suggest that the head-forward orientation is usually more practical.

Medical Conditions.   Medical conditions that might influence preference for one orientation over the other (when cross-plane positioning is not possible) are cardiopulmonary or cerebral in nature. If a cardiopulmonary condition exists that might compromise the cerebral circulation and oxygenation, being head-first and supine during takeoff and climb could increase the problem. Modest elevation of the head and the provision of increased oxygen can ameliorate the problem. The pressure that securing straps may have on the abdomen might also give some assistance. The effect of acceleration on a patient with increased intracranial pressure, being transported head-aft, can also be serious.

Acceleration cannot be modified as easily as deceleration, so the reversed forces acting on landing and braking need not be as serious as on takeoff. The head-forward position would seem preferable to the feet-forward position in cases of cerebral edema.

Conclusion.   After consideration of the factors that would influence the choice between head-forward or head-aft orientation during air transfer, the author concludes that the vast majority of cases should be transported with the head forward *if cross-plane orientation is not possible.*

The Pilot's Assistance

Circumstances having dictated a particular orientation for the patient on his stretcher, the medical flight attendant should be able to rely on the pilot to cooperate in alleviating or ameliorating the deleterious effects of various flight maneuvers. There are strict limits to how far certain maneuvers can be modified without jeopardizing the safety of the aircraft, but safe modifications can be made. When runway length is generous for the type of aircraft being used, breaking can be more gentle after landing and more runway can be used. On some occasions, acceleration for take-off may be modified if runway length is more than adequate and there are no hazards in the flight path beyond the field. Rate of climb and descent can be modified to be less severe if the extra expenditure of time is not critical.

Posture

Although F.A.A. regulations specify that passengers in aircraft must be seated with the back of the seat in the upright position and seat belts fastened during takeoff and landing, the regulations do allow a patient to be in the supine position if the medical condition does not allow the patient to be seated upright. The posture most beneficial for the patient's medical condition should be chosen, allowing for the limits imposed by the type and construction of the stretcher. Whatever the posture of the patient as he is supported on the stretcher, he must be adequately secured by straps to withstand sudden movements in *any* direction.

ENGINES RUNNING

The hazards of rotating propellers and jet-engine streams are obvious. Apart from their ability to produce direct trauma, they can propel foreign bodies into eyes and can carry sparks from lighted pipes and cigarettes to ignitable material. Engine airstreams can have a severe cooling effect when ambient temperatures are low. Therefore, special attention must be given to patients when engines are running during loading and unloading, when attention is likely to be focused elsewhere.

You may wonder why it would ever be necessary to have engines running during boarding and disembarking. There are two reasons why this may be necessary:

1. It may be essential to produce electrical power for heating and other uses, and to conserve any reservoir of battery power for future expected and unexpected use.
2. Some aircraft (mostly large aircraft) require external battery power to start the engines. Some airports may lack the motorized equipment to provide this power, so one engine must be kept running to provide the power to start the others.

Rules to be followed when approaching an aircraft which has its engines running:

1. Never approach an aircraft with engines running without an indication to do so by the pilot.

2. Always approach an aircraft from a direction that allows the pilot to see you.

Rules to be followed when approaching a helicopter:

1. Never approach the tail rotor.
2. Never approach a helicopter with engine running without an indication to do so by the pilot.
3. Always approach a helicopter from a direction that allows the pilot to see you.
4. Reduce one's walking height when approaching a helicopter with blades rotating.

There is *always danger* in approaching the tail rotor (a vertical rotor which turns the tail to the right or left by altering the direction and pitch angle of the blades). It always rotates when the main blades are rotating.

Not all helicopters have the capability of stopping the rotation of their rotor blades while the engine continues to run. Those which do not have this capability require a significant amount of time to restart the engines to operating pitch after they shut down. This should explain why patients may need to be loaded while the blades are rotating.

The height of the rotors varies with the upward thrust they are producing, and the height may be altered during an approach to the helicopter. Allowance must be made for this, and some ducking under the blades is always appropriate. Usually there is adequate safe clearance below the rotors when the helicopter is on firm, level ground. Should any special precautions need to be taken, the flight crew will direct the medical flight attendants.

Vibration and Noise

It is appropriate to mention vibration and noise with the comments related to engines running. The aviation environment is somewhat plagued by both vibration and noise, though the jet age has brought relative peace and quiet to the cabin at cruising altitudes (in some aircraft). The comfort of an executive jet cruising at 41,000 feet is hard to exceed anywhere on the ground in this noisy age of civilization.

Vibration

The sources of vibration include:

1. Engines
2. Transmission chains
3. Propellers: Primary vibrations will be in the range of 10 to 1000 Hz.
4. Multiengine beats: The engines of multiengined aircraft will only be synchronized inadvertently as regards piston firing and transmission gears. This lack of synchronization can cause regular beats of a lower frequency (1 to 10 Hz). These can be prolonged and annoying.
5. Air turbulence
6. Air movement: Over the skin of the aircraft and its protuberances. The vortices produced by propellors impinge on each other, on the airstream of flight, and on the aircraft.
7. Rotors: Rotary-winged aircraft are the main producers of noticeable

vibrations. The predominant frequencies are related to those of rotation of the blades. Other aircraft do not have the series of other accountable vibrations emanating from the vertical tail rotors or those from the unique engine train which includes the rotor head. Most of these vibrations are directly transmitted to the fuselage and its contents, including any patient or medical flight attendant. Seats and stretcher mattresses do dampen some of the vibrations. There are also external, buffeting, vibratory forces produced by the rotor blades moving the air. At low levels of flight, some of the forces are reflected from the ground and can add vibratory frequencies or increase their force. It is the noise associated with frequencies above 10 Hz that is more detrimental to the patient's care than the physiological effects of the vibrations.

8. Landing fields and taxiways: According to the nature of the surface and the speed of the aircraft, the vibrations can be coarse or fine. The coarse vibrations are more noticeable and can be annoying when attempting to write or perform a procedure.

Effects of Vibrations. Vibrations as such are not usually harmful to a patient or a medical flight attendant but can interfere with the ease of performing certain procedures such as urinary catheterization or the cannulation of a vein. Vibrations can be simple harmonic, as produced by rotors; compound harmonic from many sources, which may or may not resonate; and those from random frequencies (multiple aperiodic frequencies). In the latter, there is often a predominant frequency and this will be the one noticed. Some of these predominant frequencies may cause sporadic resonance with parts of the body. This is rarely of any clinical significance, though cases of arrhythmia and cardiac decompensation have been reported that were suspected of being due to resonating vibration.

Frequencies below those of sound (less than 10 Hz), as produced by aircraft, usually have more force than the higher frequencies. Vibrations can certainly add artifacts to a cardiac monitor screen or strip. There seems to be some physiological evidence that some vibrations induce more rapid tiring of muscles and can produce aches. Some vibrations can certainly cause an amount of stress that could hinder performance. They are annoying and can be a distraction, something a medical flight attendant must be on guard against.

Noise

The noise associated with vibration frequencies above 10 Hz is more detrimental to patients' care than the physiological effects of those vibrations. Noise, as well as the vibrations that can be felt of sensed, is a stress-producing factor that can lead to decreased human performance and more-rapid fatigue.

What is more important is that noise can interrupt communications within the cabin and in air-to-ground and air-to-air transmissions. If communications are not entirely interrupted, they can be limited by noise and thus become less accurate or misinterpreted. If hearing is difficult due to noise in the aviation environment, there can be double jeopardy when altitude has reduced audial acuity by its barometric effects on the middle ear.

With these hindrances to hearing and satisfactory communications and the headaches that can be caused by vibration, the aviation environment can be somewhat unfriendly, especially in piston-engined planes. Hints will be given later on how to ameliorate these annoyances. There have been some suggestions that subsonic vibrations (1 to 10 Hz) can cause hyperventilation, but the exact cause is obscure.

Sources of Noise.   For the most part, sources of noise are the same as the sources of vibration, with the higher-frequency components being the ones heard.

Noise from outside the plane:
1. Engines
2. Transmissions
3. Propellers and rotors
4. Jet and exhaust streams
5. Air flow outside the plane
6. Gusting of turbulent air

Noise from inside the cabin:
1. Air-conditioning
2. Pressurizing systems
3. Communications systems (useful voice and static)
4. Medical equipment in operation

Putting reputations aside, jet aircraft are generally quieter than propeller-driven aircraft at any altitude or on the tarmac. Turboprop aircraft have a different noise than those whose propellers are driven by piston engines. Turboprop engines have higher idling speeds, there are usually more blades on a propeller shaft (three or four), and the turbine exhaust has an unpleasant pitch (something like a cross between a whine and a howl).

Insulation from Noise.   The interior cabin walls are constructed with a lining of materials that absorbs some of the external noise and dampens the internal noise levels. The shape of the cabin walls is important, as any flat areas are likely to resonate with some of the frequencies of the noise and act like a sounding board. Different areas within a cabin can have very different noise levels. It is useful to know that it is noisiest in the forward area of a multiengined propeller-driven plane and is maximum in line or just behind the plane of the propellers.

Helicopter Noise.   Just as the helicopter can produce the worst vibrations of all types of aircraft, it can also produce the worst noise. A helicopter has a relatively large power train, transmission system, and noise-producing main and tail rotors. This noise is concentrated into a small cabin. Lower frequencies make for louder noise levels, and there are added external sounds from the engine exhausts that are, by necessity, close to the cabin. However, the great advantages of rotary aircraft in performance of certain missions far outway the disadvantages demonstrated by their ability to produce noise and vibrations. They will be lauded further under Helicopter Operations, later in this chapter.

Recently, changes in the design of the rotor head and the use of fiberglass for some parts of the mechanism have alleviated some of the noise inherent in rotary craft. Other innovations by the Aerospatiale Helicopter Corporation include using a polycarbonate material for the cabin hull and a rotor design which reduces blade noise.

An experimental helicopter has been flown successfully in the United States which does not have a tail rotor and uses air jets to control yaw. It is expected that this design will also reduce noise and vibration levels and eliminate the dangers of the rotating tail blades to ground personnel.

COMMUNICATIONS

The aircraft flying on an aeromedical mission needs to be able to communicate by voice with its home base. It also needs to be able to communicate with the ground telephone system so that messages may be told to a medical director, hospitals, and ground ambulance units. Likewise, the home base of operations needs to be able to communicate by voice with its aircraft.

The radio communications systems are under the control of the pilot. Communications with air traffic control centers are made using specific frequencies. The company owning or leasing the aircraft may have its own frequency so that its officers may communicate messages not concerned with the operation of the aircraft. The range of this type of transmission may not be great, and the flight crew must be monitoring the company frequency for the ground base to call its aircraft. This may not be possible when the flight crew is using other frequencies for navigational purposes.

Some aircraft have air-to-ground telephones that can be connected through the mobile department of the regional telephone companies. An aircraft so equipped can be called from a ground telephone if the telephone call sign of the aircraft is known and the mobile department can be informed of its approximate location so that the nearest relay transmitter can be used. The system sounds simple, but it is not. Whether it works at a particular time depends on many factors, including the weather and the time of day, and it is of little use on transoceanic aeromedical missions.

UNICOM

Every U.S. airport that has any radio facilities can communicate air to ground using a VHF frequency which allows line-of-sight transmission (the higher the aircraft, the longer the range). Airports with control towers have different frequencies from those that do not. A third frequency on the UNICOM system is for air-to-air communications. The system is not selective, so there is no privacy in communications. How well it will perform for a particular message will depend on how much traffic is on the frequency.

Air Traffic Control

Air traffic control radio communications are controlled by the F.A.A. (Federal Aviation Administration) in conjunction with the F.C.C. (Federal Communications Commission). A pilot filing a flight plan with A.T.C. will indicate that it is a *Lifeguard flight* if a patient is to be carried in the aircraft. This gives the pilot certain privileges, the most important of which is a better choice of altitude for the flight. This is especially important when an unpressurized aircraft is being used for the transport.

When there is a medical emergency in the air, the A.T.C. system may be utilized as a *mayday* call; in urgent cases (less than critical), an air traffic controller may pass on messages and transmit replies but not patch an air-to-ground transmission elsewhere. The use of an air traffic controller should be avoided if at all possible for any messages that are not concerned with the operation of the aircraft. The A.T.C. does become concerned with the operation of the aircraft when a medical emergency on board necessitates making an emergency landing at an airfield other than the original destination. In such cases, the controller may honor a request to communicate with any ground ambulance unit that might be required to be on the field to meet the aircraft.

ARINC

There is more sophisticated method providing air-to-ground radio communications. The company that provides that system is known as ARINC (Aeronautical Radio, Inc.), first organized in 1929 as a corporation, with the airline companies being the principal owners. Its services are now available to all aircraft operators the world over.

ARINC owns and operates a nationwide VHF air-to-ground communications network (there are 1600 VHF ground radio stations). It also provides communication service to aircraft operating over oceanic routes via long-range HF and extended-range VHF from gateway stations (New York, Houston, San Francisco, Honolulu, and San Juan). Prior arrangement must be made by an aircraft operator or a company leasing aircraft for aeromedical flights so that ARINC has a list of the personnel authorized to originate or receive CODD (central office dispatch drop) calls.

The *CODD service* is designed to provide direct voice communications between flight crews and their company operational offices via the radiotelephone frequencies controlled from ARINC centers using phone patch techniques. The frequencies are available on most aircraft radios that are used for air traffic messages and messages related to meteorological information. The frequencies are, however, different from those used for *flight safety* messages (air traffic control and meteorological). Messages that concern nonroutine matters or problems related to the crew, passengers (including patients), and cargo are known as *flight regularity* messages.

For an aircraft to receive CODD transmission via ARINC, the pilot must monitor particular frequencies by manual operation. This is not usually convenient unless specific times have been arranged for a message to be sent. If the aircraft radio is fitted with a special decoder, four preselected audio tones can activate a signal in the cockpit to alert the pilot to tune in for a message. This system is known as *SELCAL* (selective calling).

ARINC also provides another service known as *SSB LDOCF* (single-sideband long-distance operational control frequency). This system operates in the HF single-sideband suppressed carrier mode, upper sideband only. For an aircraft to use this system of communications, its radio must be compatible with the suppressed carrier mode of operation. HF transceivers designed for double-sideband operation only are not compatible. If the transceiver has both suppressed carrier mode and full carrier mode, the mode selector switch should be turned to suppressed carrier mode for ARINC communications. The suppressed carrier mode will not operate the SELCAL system to open a monitor, so the radio must have the selector switch in the full carrier mode position to receive the alerting signal. It can then be turned to the suppressed carrier mode for the message.

The ARINC communications centers have a range of frequencies they can use for transmissions, each center having the same set of frequencies. The frequencies used depend on a number of factors. In general, the higher frequencies are used during daylight hours. Whether a particular frequency will be effective to complete a transmission at a particular distance and location can depend on the time of day, local atmospheric noise, sunspot activity, and the latitude of operation.

It is expected that aircraft will use the CODD system when flying over the U.S. mainland and only use the LDOCF for international communications, but the LDOCF can be used in an emergency or if the VHF equipment is not functioning.

Air-to-Ground Radio Communications Procedures

Most air-to-ground radio channels are one-way. The equipment cannot transmit and receive at the same time, so interruptions and breakins are not possible. Voice-operated relay switches control the mode which will operate. If the ground operator and the communicator in the aircraft attempt to talk simultaneously, neither will be heard by the other.

The above facts make it important that some voice sound precedes the relevant message, so that the transmit mode is open before the message is spoken. Sounds such as "uhh," "err," or "ahem" should precede a message. The end of the message should be made clear so that the recipient of the message knows he may now reply. The words "go ahead" can be used. The word "out" should not be used unless indicating no further messages will be sent. Loud background noise in a ground station or someone talking to the radio operator over his shoulder can trip the voice-operated relay and interfere with a message being received.

When giving radio messages, speech should be firm and on an even level. Poor transmissions are not improved by shouting into the microphone. Clarity is much more important than loudness. How clear a radio message will be or how far it will travel depends on external influences as well as on the power and efficiency of the transceiver. The higher radio frequencies depend more on line of site, skip, or repeater assistance. For this reason, transmissions have a better chance of success over a long range when the aircraft is at a high altitude. Higher frequencies also work better during daylight hours.

All radio communications are influenced by sunspot activity. This activity has a cycle of intensity of about 11 years. From the radio operator's point of view, the quality of radio communications increases slowly over 7 to 8 years, then deteriorates over the next 3 years. The end of the present 8-year increase was in 1980, so the quality of communications is in the period of deterioration for another 2 years at the time of writing (1982). Irregular sunspot activity and other heavenly influences can effect transmissions at unpredictable times.

The above information should make the medical flight attendant aware of the fact that clear radio communications between the ground base and the aircraft performing a long-distance mission cannot be guaranteed at all times. This information should increase the chances of a clear message should the medical flight attendant provide the voice of transmission on the ground or in the air.

Hand-held Two-way Radios

In mission locations where there are inadequate telephone services (a permanent condition in some countries and a condition that could occur anywhere in disaster situations), two-way radios can be very useful for communications between hospitals, airports, or local operations headquarters. However, some words on their use are in order. Each country has laws governing radio transmissions. It is wise to know those laws before using two-way radios. Permission can be obtained to use them for legitimate emergency medical needs. A diplomatic consul can be helpful in this regard.

Warning
In some countries, it is a very grave offense to use transceivers without government permission, and the penalties can be harsh. In one country (at least), the penalty is execution. Consider using portable radios *only* for legitimate emergency medical needs, limit their use to an absolute minimum, and keep all messages brief and succinct.

Privacy
Radio transmissions can be over heard. Therefore, confidentialities ought to be avoided whenever possible, and the names of patients should not be identified on the air (prearranged code names can be used).

Security
Expose radio sets to the public eye as little as possible, and conceal them whenever possible—especially in countries where the penalty for improper use is death!

In the Aircraft
Portable transceivers should not be operated in a functioning aircraft as they may interfere with navigational equipment.

Electronic Cardiac Pacemakers

Avoid making radio transmissions in close proximity to patients having artificial pacemakers or wired jaws. Recently manufactured pacemakers are, however, more adequately shielded than the older models.

REFUELING

Accidents occasionally happen during refueling, and a spill of aviation fuel can occur. It is more likely to happen on smaller airfields where facilities are limited. If a spill does occur and the air is calm, fumes may contaminate the cabin. Therefore, something about the nature of the various aviation fuels should be known in order to understand the dangers involved.

Reciprocating engines (piston-driven) use a gasoline fuel known as AVGAS (in earlier days it had the more pleasant name of aviation spirit). It is a complex mixture of aliphatic and aromatic hydrocarbons with additives that can include toluene, xylene, aniline and tetraethyl lead. It comes in a number of grades somewhat equivalent to the octane levels quoted for gasolines used in automobiles.

Gas turbine engines use fuels of different types and mixtures depending on the design of the engine. Some engines can use fuels other than the recommended one for a limited number of hours if the recommended mixture is not available.

In civilian aviation in the United States, the jet fuel most commonly used is known as jet type A; a higher grade with additives is known as jet A1. In Europe and many other parts of the world, a different nomenclature is used for the fuels; jet A is equivalent to AVTUR 40/50. AVTUR comes in a variety of mixtures that might include gasoline, kerosene, high-flashpoint kerosene, aromatics, and fuel oil. The various grades have flashpoints between 110°F and 150°F. High-flashpoint kerosene is known as AVCAT in Europe and is close to what is called JP5 in the U.S. (flashpoint of 140°F). A very inflammable fuel is used to start gas turbine engines and known as AVPIN.

The hazards of aviation fuels of interest to the medical flight attendant are the risk of fire and the toxic effects of inhaling the fumes. The gasoline fuels are more volatile and have lower flashpoints, and therefore present a relatively higher risk. However, gasoline is present in many of the mixtures. Any of the fumes released by the aviation fuels are toxic if they are inhaled for any length of time. Which fuel and the length of exposure will determine the degree of toxicity or the extent of the irritation to the respiratory tract.

Inhalation of fumes and fire risks are to be avoided where possible. Therefore, it is preferable that the patient be removed from the aircraft during refueling in case a spill should contaminate the cabin. Of course, this is not always possible. A patient's medical condition or a lack of nearby facilities to accommodate him may dictate that he remain on board.

If the patient is to remain on board, the attendant must remain with him. All medical equipment that is electrically powered or has moving parts that could produce a friction spark should be turned off or disconnected. The airport authorities or the fueling agent should be informed that a patient is on board, and they should alert fire control and rescue services to be on standby.

When fuel is being pumped into an aircraft, the tanker, pumps, hose, and the aircraft are connected by grounding cables. This is a precaution against a buildup of electrostatic potential which could produce a spark. As an extra precaution, it might be the duty of the medical flight attendant to confirm that this has been done while he is responsible for the patient in the aircraft.

While it is obvious that there should be no smoking in or near the aircraft during refueling, thought should be given to the distance that the wind, propeller, and jet streams can carry sparks. The usual recommendation is that there should be no smoking within 50 feet of an aircraft on the ground, but 100 feet might be more appropriate.

OTHER MISSION CONSIDERATIONS

Distance

The traveling distance of the mission is, of course, of considerable importance and limits the choice of aircraft to those that have an adequate range and fuel capacity. This is especially so when missions of over 1000 miles are being contemplated. In many cases, aircraft that have a long range and the necessary higher speed need longer runways. If the facilities from which the patient is to be dispatched and received respectively do not have airports capable of allowing a long-range aircraft to land because of runway or other conditions, other arrangements must be made for the transfer of the patient to airports that can accept the long-range craft.

Range

The range of an aircraft may be longer than the distance it must travel between the dispatching and the receiving facilities. However, if it is ascertained that refueling services are not available at the distant end of the mission, the range must be long enough to make both legs of the mission or refueling stops must be made elsewhere. It is in the patient's interest to avoid refueling stops whenever possible.

Airports and Airstrips

These must be matched to the type of aircraft being used. It is obvious that if the runway length is not sufficient for the plane, it cannot be used.

The facilities available at the airport must also be considered. These would include: fueling abilities, abilities to replenish supplies, sanitary arrangements as per health codes, freedom from insect disease vectors, custom and immigration clearances, and acceptable water supplies (see International Missions).

Takeoff and Landing Lengths

These have already been mentioned; however, it should be noted that although these are closely related to the type of aircraft used, they can under marginal conditions be related to the load carried and the weather and climatic conditions. The margins of safety dictate which airports can or cannot be used under emergency conditions.

Proximity of the Dispatching and Receiving Facilities to the Airport

Planes that can fly faster and longer usually need longer runways and more sophisticated airports. When long-distance flights are necessary, the choice of planes is limited to those with the appropriate range, assuming speed is important and hops can be avoided. When short- or medium-distance missions are planned (less than 750 miles), it does not seem sensible to choose an aircraft capable of great speed but that must land at an airport a great distance from the facility that will dispatch and receive the patient. One hour saved in the air can be offset by an uncomfortable 45-minute ground ambulance ride before or after the flight.

Cruising Speed

Knowing the cruising speed of the aircraft indicates to the flight attendant how long the patient will be airborne and allows him to calculate the estimated time of arrival, to notify the ground transport that will meet the plane and the receiving facility, and to judge the amount of supplies required, especially oxygen requirements for longer flights.

Payload

A light aircraft is severely limited in the load it can carry. Therefore, when a light aircraft must be used for an aeromedical evacuation, the payload must be accurately known in order to know what personnel and equipment can accompany the patient. Whether a friend or relative can accompany the patient must be judged with payload in mind. The amount of oxygen that might be required to be carried also alters the load considerably. (See Oxygenation in Part III for the weight of oxygen cylinders.) In addition, the load a plane can carry is intimately related to the distance it might have to travel, its fuel capacity, and the terrain it must traverse.

Climates

It is often surprising how quickly one can fly from one climate to another. This can occur in both an east-west and a north-south direction. The majority of aircraft have air-conditioning systems that can adequately keep the cabin at a comfortable temperature. What must be considered is the capability of the aircraft to maintain that comfort during stopovers. Many aircraft of the light variety lose all power when the engines are shut down. It can be imagined what might happen to the temperature of the cabin in arctic or equatorial regions during stopovers of any length of time. Therefore, if severe climatic conditions are expected, a plane having internal power independent of the driving engines must be used or arrangements must be made to move the patient to climatized accommodations during the time the engines are shut down.

In the unlikely event that the heating system of an aircraft fails in flight, the temperature outside the aircraft will determine the cooling of the cabin as the insulating qualities of the fuselage and cabin walls are defeated. The temperature outside the aircraft can be roughly estimated by subtracting 2°C for every thousand feet the plane is above the ground temperature. For example, if the ground temperature is 10°C and the altitude is 15,000 feet, the temperature outside the plane will be 30°C below that of the ground (−20°C). If the cabin temperature is 24°C (75°F), the differential between cabin and the outside will be 44°C. Unless the plane loses altitude or the heating system is made to work again, blankets will be urgently needed.

Terrain

It should be obvious that a pressurized aircraft is required to traverse mountains over 10,000 feet high. A mission that must be flown over large areas of water must be equipped with escape and safety devices adequate to cope with a forced landing on water.

Types of Fuel

All major airports have all types of fuel that might be needed to refuel an aircraft turning round on a mission or hopping through. This is not necessarily true at smaller airports, and it must be known if refueling facilities with the correct type of fuel are available should a refueling stop need to be made. This is primarily the concern of the captain of the aircraft, but it can be of concern to a medical flight attendant should a mission be flown to an out-of-the-way place on an emergency basis. (See Refueling earlier in this Part for a description of the different types of fuel.)

International Permits

Aircraft may be chartered for use in an aeromedical evacuation from a foreign country. In such cases, it must be ascertained that the aircraft charter company has the necessary documents that give its aircraft permission to fly to the destinated country. Attempting to arrange such documentation on an emergency basis can cause considerable delays and may prevent a successful evacuation if the time element is critical.

Pressurization

The cabin altitude pressures to be expected at various altitudes in different aircraft will be discussed under Modifications of Care in Part 3.

In an unpressurized aircraft, the pressure in the cabin is, of course, equivalent to that of the altitude of the aircraft above sea level. Above 10,000 feet, supplemental oxygen is required by air crew members to ensure adequate physical and mental capability. This assumes that the physical exercise will be limited to lever pulling, button pushing, and wheel turning. A medical flight attendant may need to perform more physical exercise than the cockpit crew, such as lifting and posturing the patient and moving about the cabin to move and use equipment. Therefore, his need for supplementary oxygen may exceed that of the flight crew. The patient may have a definite need for a higher concentration of supplemental oxygen. Gaseous expansion with altitude can limit what the patient can tolerate according to the medical conditions he suffers.

Access

The size and position of access doors are always important, but more so when it comes to loading a patient on a Stryker orthopedic frame or other stretcher with extra attachments. It can be embarrassing to arrive with a patient at the door of an aircraft and then find that the stretcher or frame to which the patient is attached will not fit through the door (see Loading and Unloading).

Cabin Space

It is no less embarrassing to have the stretcher fit through the aircraft door and then find that there is not enough room in the cabin to accommodate the patient and his accoutrements. The height of the cabin makes certain procedures on patients very difficult. However, there are ways to overcome the lack of height that reduces the pressure head in IV reservoirs (see Intravenous Therapy).

The cabin space and seats available dictate the number of relatives and friends that can accompany the patient, if not already limited by the payload. In deciding whether others accompany the patient, space is one consideration, but the seriousness of the patient's condition and what might need to be done for him during the flight are of more importance. Some procedures (especially bloody ones) are difficult to perform with relatives breathing down the medical attendant's neck. The payload may often be used as the excuse for excluding relatives from the flight when it is in the patient's interest.

Electrical Harness

On international missions when foreign aircraft may be chartered, the voltage of any electrical harness must be known. It could be 6, 12, 110, or 230 volts and may not be compatible with the equipment to be supplied. The voltage may be correct, but the configuration of the sockets and plugs may not be compatible. The cyclic period of an alternating current may also be incompatible with the equipment to be used. Because of this and the fact that many aircraft do not have the necessary outlets, battery-powered equipment is desirable and spare batteries need to be carried. Batteries should not be of the liquid variety that could leak their corrosive contents.

Auxiliary Services—Oxygen Outlets and Suction Inlets

It is a great luxury to be able to use an aircraft which is dedicated to aeromedical use and has installed oxygen outlets and suction inlets. However, the capability of these services must not be taken for granted, and the amount of oxygen and the possible flow rates should be known. The time/use limitations of these services should be estimated before a mission is flown without backup supplies of oxygen and portable battery-driven suction apparatus.

Amphibians

There are some missions that could best be performed using amphibious aircraft. Consideration should be given to their use when their versatility is desirable and there are suitable arrangements for the transfer of the patient to ground transport from a mooring or landing dock. Some of the fixed-wing amphibians have very desirable cabin space and safety features when used over large tracts of water. However, the leaway on landing runs is somewhat offset by the disadvantages associated with tidal and wave conditions and limitations in servicing and refueling facilities.

Safety Margins for Conditions that Might Be Encountered

All aircraft are not capable of flying safely in adverse weather conditions. Those that can are termed "all-weather aircraft." The urgency with which a mission must be flown might place limitations on how long a flight might be postponed to wait for favorable weather and climatic conditions. In such a case, an aircraft capable of weathering a variety of adverse conditions might be chosen over one which does not have such a capability. Much depends on the sophistication of the navigational and landing-assist equipment installed in the aircraft and on the rating of the pilot in command. On a more somber note, some aircraft are more vulnerable than others to gunfire, and not all missions will be flown from militarily safe areas.

In emergency situations, the only available runway may not be the recommended length from a safety point of view, but it must be used. Aircraft are capable of braking more severely than usual, and this may allow landing on a shorter runway. When runway runs out and the brakes are not going to stop the aircraft before disaster, there are maneuvers (uncomfortable and somewhat dangerous) that can swing the plane around suddenly and limit further forward movement.

Rescue and Escape Appliances

In the operation manuals of all aircraft are the directives for operation should a forced landing on water or land be necessary. A medical flight attendant should be conversant with these instructions. This is possibly best accomplished by being briefed by the pilot, which ensures that the pilot is up to date with these instructions for the type of aircraft he is flying.

Aerovac Experience of the Flight Crew

There has to be close cooperation and coordination between the flight crew and the medical flight attendant. The flight crew must be used to assist in the loading and unloading of the patient and making him secure in the cabin, and to generally assist in the care of the patient.

If the plane is flown with minimal disturbance to the comfort of the patient, it can mean the difference between good and bad care during the flight. The attitude and personal relationship of the pilot and other members of the flight crew toward the patient and those accompanying him can also make a great deal of difference to the comfort and confidence of the patient. A flight crew with previous experience at aeromedical evacuation is more likely to have the necessary attributes to cooperate in a manner most beneficial to the welfare of the patient.

Availability

Compromises have to be made. The choice of aircraft to accomplish a mission will often depend on what is available, and it will rarely be ideal for its task. Improvisation may be necessary to make up for deficiencies the aircraft may have in its ability to provide the service required. This is where the talents of the medical flight attendant must flourish.

When there is a strict limitation on the aircraft available, a decision has to be made whether to use a given aircraft or to use other means to care for the patient (i.e., ground transport or leave the patient where he is). Risks must be balanced, but knowing the capabilities of the aircraft being offered makes for a logical decision.

Table 7. Approximate Aircraft Charter Rates (1982).[a]

Aircraft Type	Approx. Cruising Speed (mph)	No. of Stretcher Patients	Hourly Flight Cost	Waiting Time (Hourly Cost)
6-Passenger executive jet	250 to 400	1 (sometimes 2)	750–1200	75–100
18-Passenger high-performance twin turboprop	170 to 250	Up to 3	600–850	75–90
8-Passenger pressurized twin	150 to 230	1	250–350	30–45
5-Passenger unpressurized twin	120 to 200	1	200–300	25–35

[a] Prices in U.S. dollars.

Note: As waiting times are rarely estimated accurately, a charter company will usually give a quote for the proposed mission with a specified number of waiting hours above which extra hourly charges will accrue.

Table 8.   Other Mission Costs.

1. General operating costs of the aircraft based on hours flown and waiting times
2. Fuel
3. Airport expenses: landing fees, supplies and services, parking fees. The latter can be expensive in some countries, and some South American countries have been known to arbitrarily change the fees according to the origin of the aircraft and have recently charged as much as $600 to park overnight.
4. Ground ambulance expenses at point of pickup, arrival, and occasionally at a stopover location
5. Flight crew
6. Medical flight crew
7. Bed and board for flight crew and medical attendants
8. Medications and oxygen
9. Medical equipment: respiratory, suction, IVs, monitor/defibrillator, orthopedic traction devices, special stretcher, catheters, and drainage systems
10. Bedpans, urinals, sheets and blankets, etc.
11. Nutritional items for patients and crew
12. Telephone and radio communications
13. Visa and immunization expenses
14. Personal airport taxes
15. Other ground transportation expenses
16. Miscellaneous expenses which always arise

$15,000 is not an unusual amount for an international aeromedical mission for the transfer of one patient.

Cost

Unfortunately, cost must always be taken into consideration. It would be nice if this was not so and an aircraft could be chosen for a mission solely on its suitability. Transport of a single patient by air is still an expensive business on a long haul. However, many medium- and short-range missions can be cost-effective relative to ground transport and can often be more comfortable, quicker, and safer for the patient.

Compromises have to be made, and speed and some comfort may have to be sacrificed to some extent in order to make a mission financially feasible but still beneficial for the patient. The specifics of a medical insurance contract sometimes dictate what can be provided for a patient with respect to aeromedical transport. It is pleasing to report that many insurance programs that cover repatriation by air for medical reasons are becoming available for travelers.

Over long distances (transcontinental and transoceanic), medical transfer by commercial scheduled airlines is usually less expensive than chartering a plane privately. It is also likely to be a more comfortable way of flying: nutritional needs can be easily met, toilet facilities are present, and adequate space can be present. However, this means of medical transfer is still expensive relative to traveling as a regular passenger (see Transfer of Patients by Scheduled Commercial Airlines).

For those unfamiliar with air chartering, rough price ranges for some types of aircraft may give some indication of the expenses involved in medical air transport (see Table 7). When estimating the total cost of an aeromedical mission, other important mission costs must also be considered (see Table 8).

HELICOPTER OPERATIONS

The helicopter frequently exceeds the fixed-wing aircraft in the production of noise and vibration. These are minor disadvantages in comparison with the many advantages of rotary craft. Their ability to land in small areas away from airfields and quickly carry patients to the doorstep of a medical facility often eliminates the need for ground ambulances. They can save a significant amount of transport time and avoid multiple transfers. Being able to hover allows a helicopter to perform unique functions in rescue work. Patients have been rescued from mountainsides, mountaintops, crevasses, high buildings, seas, and lakes.

Most helicopters have an endurance range of between 300 and 500 miles. As most medical missions do not provide an opportunity to refuel at the pickup point, this means that the range of operations is usually between 150 and 250 miles. Cruising speeds are between 110 and 150 miles per hour.

The rotor blades of these aircraft have a diameter between 30 and 40 feet. Very few helicopters have the ability to stop the main blades from rotating without shutting down the engines. Some do have brakes to the main rotor that can slow the rotation considerably during ground operations. The rotating blades can have a cooling effect and can cause the movement of dust and dirt particles during loading and unloading. A properly surfaced and located helipad reduces dust problems.

The various helicopters suitable for aeromedical work are listed in Table 9.

Landing Area Requirements

1. Minimum of 100 feet in diameter.
2. No hazards within 200 feet. Hazards include buildings, overhead wires, poles, lamp standards, and tall trees.
3. No loose debris within 200 feet.
4. Level ground.
5. Ground wind direction indicator 100 feet from the center of the landing area. A wind indicator can be a windsock, improvised flag, or a smoke grenade. Smoke grenades should only be used downwind of the landing area.

Table 9. Helicopters Adaptable as Air Ambulances.

	C	RD	MUL	R	S	A	AC
Single Engine							
Bell JetRanger III	3	33.3	1584	340	134	13,500	300
Hughes 500 D	3	26.4	1380	320	162	15,000	310
Bell LongRanger II	4 (2)	37.0	1948	350	130	19,500	450
Aerospatiale A Star (France)	4	35.1	1940	410	138	15,000	430
Alouette 3 (SA 316 B)	4	36.2	2300	360	120	20,000	?
Twin Engines							
Aerospatiale Twin Star (France)	4 (2)	35.1	2263	400	145	14,800	680
Bell 222	5 (2)	39.8	2990	420	153	12,800	2000
Agusta 109 All (Italy)	4 (2)	36.1	2090	420	161	15,000	1100
MBB B0105 CBS (Germany)	4 (2)	32.2	2511	370	143	17,000	800
Sikorsky S 76	5 (2)	44.0	4700	580	164	15,000	1700
Aerospatiale Dauphin 2 (France)	5 (2)	39.1	4176	580	170	15,000	1800

	C	RD	MUL	R	S	A	AC
Bell 212	6 (2)	48.0	5057	225	113	14,200	1200
Bell 412	6 (2)	46.0	5333	240	140	20,000	1900
Bell 214 ST	8 (3)	52.0	7987	460	155	?	4500

Codes for Table 9

C — Carrying capacity. Includes one stretcher patient. Does not include flight deck crew. The number below in parentheses indicates the number of stretcher patients that could be carried with in-flight care.

RD — Diameter of main rotor blades (feet).

MUL — Maximum useful load (lbs).

R — Range in statute miles (endurance hours × normal cruising speed).

S — Normal cruising speed (statute miles per hour). Craft can fly faster. Block time not applicable except for engine start and runup time.

A — Altitude service ceiling.

AC — Approximate cost of new aircraft (in thousands of U.S. dollars).

Identification of Landing Areas

A helicopter requested to pick up a patient from a hard-to-pinpoint area will need some assistance from those at the pickup site. Flashing lights of emergency vehicles can attract the pilot. Colored smoke grenades can also be used if they are carefully placed downwind. At night, the flashing lights of emergency vehicles are again useful. If the headlights of vehicles are used, the vehicle should be 100 feet downwind with the headlights illuminating the landing area. As soon as it is felt that the headlights are no longer of advantage to the pilot (i.e., when the helicopter has identified the landing zone and is using its own headlights), the vehicle lights should be turned off so as not to effect the vision of the pilot.

Placement and Orientation

Whenever possible, patients should be transported in a cross-cabin orientation, forward in the cabin. Most helicopter maneuvers are in a nose-down attitude of 10° to 15°. The patient is more secure and more easily attended if he is forward of the attendant.

3

AEROMEDICAL CARE

MODIFICATIONS OF CARE

Taxiing

The noise within an aircraft is maximum while its engines are running on the ground, especially during engine runup (testing the engines before takeoff). As the plane is taxiing, there is the added noise of the wheels on the ground. Within the cabin, if it is not separated from the cockpit by a closed door, the noise of radio communications will be added.

The patient's condition and temperament might suggest that he be protected from the noise by muffs, soft earplugs, or by a scarf or towel over the ears. Complete protection is hardly possible and is not desirable, as the attendant must be able to communicate with the patient. Measurements of vital signs, other observations, and adjustments of oxygenation or fluid therapy equipment should be made before taxiing begins. They can be made during taxiing but with more difficulty due to the noise and the vibrations. Recheck the securing of the patient, passengers, and equipment.

Takeoff

The medical flight attendant must be seated and belted during takeoff. This limits what attention can be given to the patient by physical means. It should not limit physical contact by touch nor the ability to verbalize reassurance and to give advice on how to ameliorate ear and sinus pressure. Remember that the attention of the flight deck crew must not be distracted during takeoff by events in the cabin.

Climb

During initial climbout, the angle of climb might be steep, and some turbulence should be anticipated. The flight attendant must be seated and belted, but always ready to assist the patient should airsickness develop.

The patient should be advised on methods of clearing the eustachian tubes during ascent. As altitude is gained, the air in the middle ear expands. It does not always equalize of its own accord and is held up by eustachian obstruction. Since air is trying to get *out* of the middle ear during ascent, a Valsalva maneuver should not be used (i.e., holding the nose, closing the mouth, and increasing pressure in the oronasal pharynx). Moving the jaw from side to side with the mouth open is often successful in relieving the pressure. Some persons can voluntarily close the mouth and glottis and produce a negative pressure in the pharynx by depressing the structures that comprise the floor of the mouth. It only takes a little practice, and this method could be taught to the patient during taxiing.

If eustachian obstruction is known or expected from examination of the patient before the flight, a nasal spray [Afrin (oxymetazoline hydrochloride 0.05%)] can be tried. Two or three sniffs up each nostril is usually sufficient, and the effects may last many hours. Chewing and swallowing have been recommended for eustachian obstruction. Children can be given lollipops to suck on, but this may increase the amount of swallowed air. This is not often of any serious consequence, but it could be if a sick patient has an abdominal illness and already is gaseous.

As the climb becomes more gentle and smooth, the attendant's seatbelt can be unfastened—with the pilot's permission. (The pilot may be aware that more turbulence is to be expected shortly.) When the movements of the aircraft allow it, vital signs should be checked against the preflight measurements. The adequacy of oxygenation should be checked as per respiratory comfort, depth, and rate; skin color; and changes in cerebration. This would also be the time to consult a portable altimeter and tape it somewhere in the cabin where it can be seen at any time. The instrument should have been set at takeoff field altitude as a reference. Intravenous flows should be frequently monitored and adjusted as necessary, and some estimation should be made of when a reservoir might be depleted. If a cardiac monitor is connected to the patient, this would be the time to check the leads, arrange them to obtain the fewest artifacts, and operate the writeout as a test strip to compare with a previous tracing. If the monitor has multilead capability, each fixed lead should be tried to obtain the most informative one.

Turns

It is during and after turns that the patient may lose his orientation. If a ground or cloud horizontal reference is not visible, the inner ear may provide false information, and vertigo leading to nausea and vomiting can occur. The patient should be advised not to make sudden movements of the head and to dimly watch an outside reference point if this is practical. The same advice should be followed by the attendant.

Descent

Descent is often more uncomfortable than climb with regard to both the rate of pressure changes and their effects on physiology, and to experiencing patchy turbulence. Descent can be divided into three periods:

1. Initial and prolonged: loss of altitude to prepare for landing.
2. Approach legs: direction changes while maneuvering to landing approach.
3. Final approach: final descent to touch down.

Initial Descent
As soon as the aircraft begins to lose altitude from its cruising level, cabin pressure can begin to increase (even in pressurized aircraft). Pressure stabilization of the middle ear becomes a concern shortly thereafter.

The rate of pressure change is usually greater in descent than in ascent. The effect on the ears is also greater because of the anatomy of the eustachian tube which acts as a valve that allows air to pass out of the middle ear easier than it can return. As the air in the middle ear reduces in volume during descent, a negative pressure can develop, drawing-in the tympanic membrane and causing considerable pain. A similar state of affairs can occur with the facial sinuses, especially the frontal sinuses when there is a degree of congestion around the ostia. The pain can be excruciating. Fortunately, the frequent gentle use of the Valsalva maneuver can force air back into the middle ears and the sinuses. The person performing this maneuver knows it has been successful by the sound of a not-unpleasant whistle as the air enters the middle ear.

If it has been more than 4 hours since a nasal spray was used, it could also be used if indicated. Rocking the jaw also helps, as it does during ascent. This maneuver alters the angle of the eustachian tubes to fortuitously give them the maximum caliber at one point during the movement of the jaw.

Attention to trapped air in the ear and sinuses should continue until after the plane has landed. Much more needs to be attended to during the initial descent, as the maneuvering to approach and the final approach of the flight make certain procedures difficult and temporarily incapacitate the medical flight attendant. The pilot should therefore give warning when the aircraft is about to descend. This will give the medical flight attendant the opportunity to check and recheck the patient's condition, complete medical records, tidy and secure all equipment that has been used in a portable manner, and generally prepare the patient for his transfer from the aircraft to ground transport on landing. It is also the time when it might be appropriate to have the pilot send a radio message to confirm arrangements for the ground transport to meet the flight. The same radio communication may give information on the weather conditions to be expected at the airport, and the patient can be dressed or draped to suit those conditions. (See Intravenous Therapy later in this Part for information on control of IV flow during descent.)

Approach Legs
As the aircraft nears the landing field, it may be necessary for it to make a number of turns to maneuver into the final approach path. These turns are usually made at altitudes where the worst near-ground turbulent air can rock and bounce the aircraft. The security of the patient and the flight attendant's own seatbelt must be attended to before the turbulent part of the flight is reached.

Final Approach
Toward the end of the final approach just before touch down, deceleration forces come into play and rapidly increase in some large aircraft or in fast, light jets, thus reducing the length of the ground roll. The patient and the attendant must be braced for the deceleration and must expect increased noise at touch down.

Landing
The moments just before landing often generate a high degree of anxiety for both the medical flight attendant and the patient. The attendant can lighten the anxiety by talking to the patient through the noise, explaining how he will be transferred to his destination.

Turbulence

The bumpy variety of air turbulence at low altitudes is predominantly caused by the *uneven heating of the earth's surface* and the structures on it. Large wooded areas and water surfaces absorb heat, other surfaces reflect heat, and still others produce heat. As this turbulent air near to the ground rises, it becomes more stable. The altitude at which relatively calm air will be found varies from time to time and from day to day. With hot ground temperatures, calm air may not be found until above 6000 to 8000 feet.

Most turbulence is associated with the *air currents around cloud formations*. Clouds are rarely present over 40,000 feet, which offers little consolation to those flying missions at much lower altitudes in light aircraft. However, the turbulence associated with clouds is predictable to a certain extent. Meteorological reports and en route reports of other flyers can inform the pilot where to expect turbulence. Routes and altitudes can be chosen to avoid the turbulence. If it cannot be avoided, the medical flight attendant will at the very least be briefed on its likelihood so he can be prepared to meet it.

A third type of turbulence is known as *"clear air turbulence."* This can be present at altitudes up to, but rarely above, 30,000 feet. Clear air turbulence might be caused by the vagaries of moving air masses of different atmospheric pressures or temperatures, uneven heating by solar or other radiations, and sometimes by persisting effects of the vortices produced by other aircraft. It is not possible to accurately predict where clear air turbulence will be found or how severe it will be. Reports from other pilots who have located areas of clear air turbulence may assist others in avoiding it. When an area with this turbulence is entered and it is disturbing enough to warrant avoidance, altitude can be changed to a smoother one.

A medical flight attendant should not expect immediate change in altitude (that is, a change under the control of the pilot) as soon as clear air turbulence is encountered. It must be flown through for a certain length of time to judge its extent. Changing altitude can alter airspeed, diminish range, and impinge on fuel reserves. Therefore, it is preferable to avoid altitude change on a long haul when the optimum height and cruising speed have been attained.

Changing altitude means the medical flight attendant has to consider the changes in atmospheric pressure that might occur in the cabin. Unfortunately, the modification in care when the aircraft is in turbulent air is toward less-detailed care of the patient with regard to taking of vital signs, giving medications, and adjusting oxygen and fluid intake. The primary concern of the attendant is to ensure the patient's safety by being properly secured and being prepared to assist the patient as well as possible from a secured seat should he vomit.

This can be difficult, but the attendant must be seated and belted in a fixed seat. It should be noted that some temporary seats in some aircraft have folding backs that must be properly latched or otherwise secured. An injured medical flight attendant is of little use to a sick or injured patient. Therefore, the attendant must take every precaution to be properly secured during the passage through turbulent air. Likewise, an airsick attendant is a detriment to good patient care, and he must be prepared to take some precautions to limit the chances of it occurring. (See Airsickness later in this Part for precautions.)

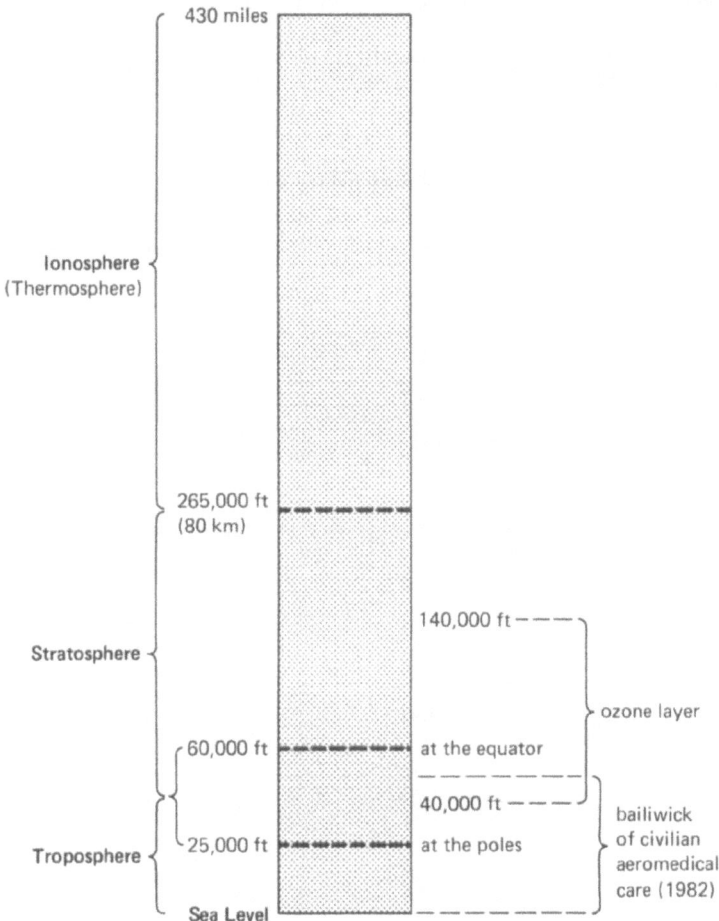

Figure 23.   Layers of the atmosphere.

Altitude

The Atmosphere
For an enlightened understanding of the effects of altitude on the human body, especially on that of an ill or injured patient, some basic knowledge of the earth's atmosphere is necessary. In this space age, aviation medicine is concerned with layers of the atmosphere above those used during aeromedical missions. It will not be long before an aeromedical evacuation from space might be necessary. The success of the space shuttle program has made a space evacuation more feasible.

Aviation medicine is already concerned with the environment beyond the earth's atmosphere, and man's exploration of space has depended on the ability of aviation medicine to protect him in that environment.

The atmosphere is conveniently divided into concentric layers according to the thermal features of each layer (Figs. 23 and 24). Nearest to the earth's surface is the *troposphere*, in which the majority of medical missions will be flown. Many will be flown above this layer in the stratosphere.

The troposphere has an uneven height to its upper boundary, as its height depends on the surface and air temperatures below it that are produced by solar energy. The intensity of the temperatures depends on

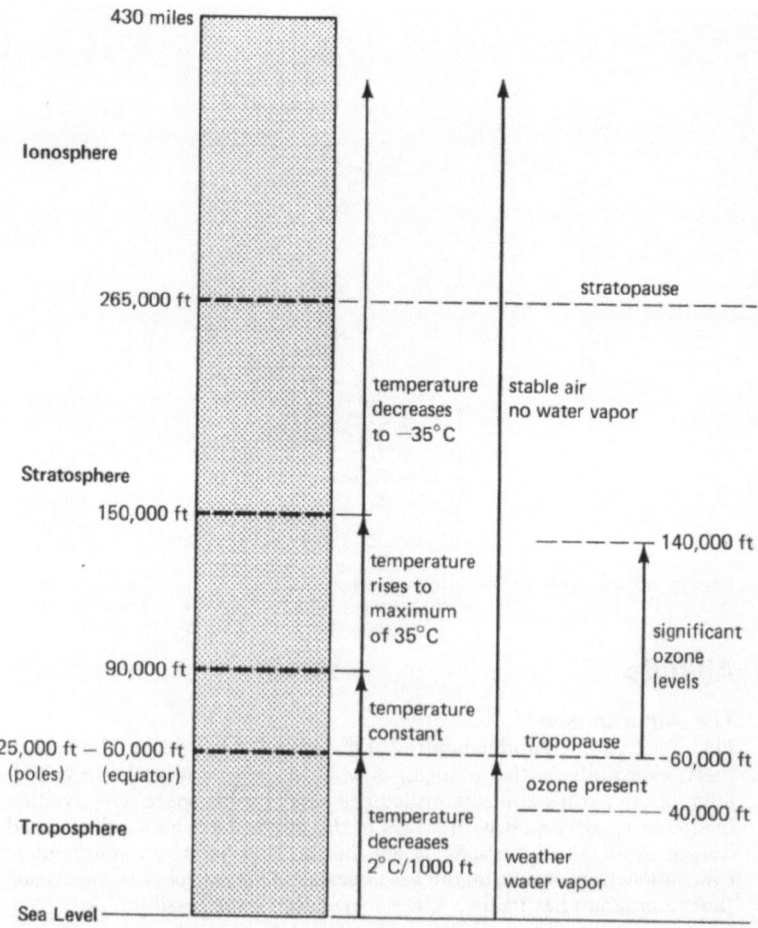

Figure 24.   Characteristics of atmospheric layers.

Table 10. Composition of the Atmosphere.

Gas	Volume	Percent[a]
Oxygen	20.95	21
Nitrogen	78.09	78
Argon	0.93	1
Carbon dioxide	0.03	3
Neon	1.8×10^{-3}	
Helium	5.2×10^{-4}	Insignificant? Yet
Krypton	1.1×10^{-4}	mysteriously significant!
Xenon	8.7×10^{-6}	
Hydrogen	5×10^{-5}	

[a] Useful approximations.

the axis the earth presents to the sun. The upper boundary of the troposphere is approximately 60,000 feet at the equator (a height rarely flown on medical missions except in advanced military aircraft). The boundary with the stratosphere is only approximately 25,000 feet at the poles. In higher latitudes, many medical air transfers will be flown in the stratosphere using pressurized aircraft.

Composition of the Atmosphere (Table 10). The composition of the atmosphere does not vary to any appreciable extent with altitude. For practical purposes, each component of the atmosphere is diminished to the same extent with altitude. Most of the small variation present in air at low altitudes is man-caused; an increase in carbon monoxide from cities, factories, engines, stoves, and smokers.

We on earth rely on the ozone layer to screen out harmful levels of ultraviolet radiation. Ironically, ozone is extremely toxic at more intimate levels (10 parts per million can be lethal). Advanced aircraft flying in the ozone layer of the stratosphere cannot compress the outside air (what little there is of it) for pressurization of the cabin. The heat generated to attain the enormous compression required of the thin air and the presence of ozone would have to be compensated for. Future medical flight attendants might be interested to learn that vitamins E and C may provide some protection against damage due to inhalation of toxic levels of ozone.[2]

The Troposphere

Characteristics of the Troposphere

1. Presence of weather and turbulence
2. Temperature decreases with altitude
3. Water vapor is present
4. Composition of the atmosphere is constant
5. Atmospheric pressure decreases with altitude

[2] From Melton, C. E. Effects of long-term exposure to low levels of ozone: A review. Aviat. Space Environ. Med. 53(2):105–111, 1982.

If an aircraft has the ability to cruise above the troposphere, it can avoid some of the problems that weather and turbulence provide. At these altitudes there is less strain on the aircraft, those on board, and the fuel supply. In the troposphere, temperature falls with altitude at a mean lapse rate of approximately 2°C for each 1000 feet of altitude gained and continues to do so until the top of the troposphere is reached. If the temperature on the ground below the aircraft is known, a rough estimate can be made of the temperature outside the aircraft, assuming the altitude is known. There is obviously a need for an efficient heating system for the cabin. It is unlikely that such a system will fail, but for that and other reasons a supply of blankets should be carried on all missions to all climatic areas of the world.

Water Vapor. The lower the temperature of an air mass, the less its capacity for holding water vapor. The capacity decreases with altitude until its presence is, for all intents and purposes, absent above the tropopause (the junction of the troposphere and the stratosphere). This is of some practical importance in pressurized aircraft which have a system that compresses air from outside the aircraft. If there is no system working to humidify the air that has been compressed, the air will become progressively drier with altitude. The recirculation of the air for ventilation purposes dries it further. This adds to the importance of properly humidifying therapeutic oxygen when it is being administered. The oxygen stored in cylinders under pressure for use in the aviation environment has to be very dry to prevent blockage of outlets and lines with freezing.

The Stratosphere
The stratosphere starts at the boundary of the troposphere (the tropopause). At this boundary, the temperature ceases to drop with altitude gain, and it remains relatively constant with *vertical* altitude change. The upper boundary of the stratosphere was designated when it was thought that the temperatures were relatively constant to a height of 265,000 feet (80 km), the arbitrary height of the stratopause (the junction of the stratosphere with the thermosphere). It has since been learned that above 90,000 feet (30 km) temperature increases progressively to 150,000 feet (50 km) then decreases progressively to the outermost boundary of the stratosphere with the thermosphere.

Characteristics of the Stratosphere

1. Weather is absent.
2. No change in temperature with altitude (in altitudes used for aeromedical flights).
3. Lack of water vapor.
4. Ozone present (from 60,000 to 150,000 feet).
5. Atmospheric pressure continues to decrease with altitude.

The Thermosphere (Ionosphere)
Above the stratosphere is the thermosphere. The thermosphere extends from 265,000 feet to 430 miles above the earth. It has a progressive rise in temperature with altitude to almost 2000°C. This layer is also known as the ionosphere, as the particles present are charged as electrons and ions.

Independent Life-Support Cabin

At very high altitudes, the air is too thin to permit sufficient compression to pressurize the cabin. An independent life-support cabin must be used which has the internal capability of controlling the pressure from stored or generated gases, with control of the composition of the cabin air. A method of absorbing excess carbon dioxide needs to be provided.

Environmental Atmospheric Pressures on Aeromedical Flights

Before considering the various physiological effects of a decreased atmospheric pressure and the effects of changes in those pressures associated with climb and descent, a knowledge of what those pressures might be is essential. In *unpressurized aircraft*, the pressure in the cabin will be the same as the ambient pressure (outside the aircraft), which depends on the altitude (Fig. 25). Note that the pressure is approximately halved at

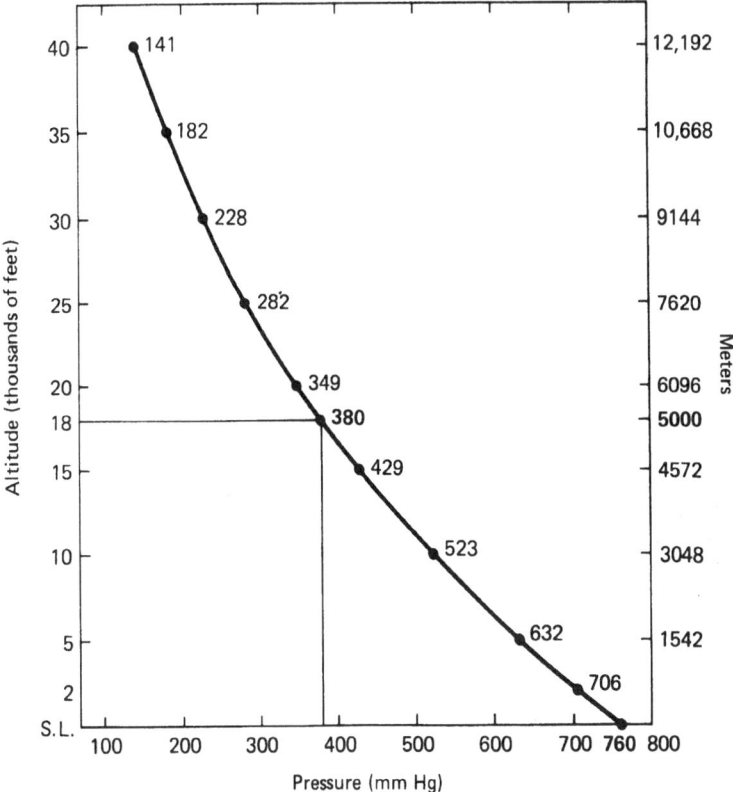

Figure 25.   Pressure reduction with altitude. Based on the international standard atmosphere which specifies mean temperature lapse rate from a mean sea level temperature where the pressure is 760 mm Hg, gravitational acceleration is constant, and the tropopause is 36,089 feet at latitude 40° north.

5000 meters or 18,000 feet. There are a number of reasons, but 5000 meters has always been of considerable importance and enchantment to mountaineers.

Pressurized Aircraft

What the pressure will be at different altitudes in a pressurized cabin will be determined by the efficiency of the pressurizing equipment (i.e., the compressor, cooler, and excess pressure vent), the number of potential leaks for the pressure, and the pressure differential that the fuselage can safely tolerate. Some high-performance aircraft can maintain sea level pressure over 20,000 feet. A Falcon 20 is reputed to be able to maintain sea level pressure to 23,000 feet. Such high-performance planes will be flying above this level when used for patient transfer, so a sea level atmosphere cannot be expected for the patient. In fact, the majority of pressurized aircraft do not maintain sea level pressure at any appreciable altitude.

Table 11 lists the altitude measurements that were taken with a portable altimeter on two scheduled flights. These measurements give some indication of how pressures decrease in the cabin with altitude and the rates of those changes.

High-performance executive jets are frequently used for medical transfers of distances over 1000 miles. The three best-known jets are the Gates Learjet, the Cessna Citation, and the Dassault-Breguet Falcon. At altitudes above 40,000 feet, where they will economically fly, a cabin altitude of 8000 feet is to be expected.

Rate of Climb/Descent

In unpressurized aircraft there is a lack of protection against the decreasing pressure as altitude is gained. The rate of decrease is relative (directly) to the rate of climb of the aircraft. Many unpressurized aircraft have the ability to climb more than 1000 feet per minute. This may often require modification by the pilot to a more gradual climb, as many patients will not tolerate this rate of pressure change. On the other hand, a pressurized aircraft may climb at a rate well over 1000 feet per minute, but the relative rate of climb in the cabin will be much less. Table 11 shows that the cabin rate of climb is between 200 and 300 feet per minute and the rate of descent is approximately 400 feet per minute but these rates fluctuate at different altitudes. The changes in rate of descent are often due to the pilot following the instructions of air traffic control. They can also be influenced by instrument landing operations.

Limitation of Pressurization

The limits to pressurization depend mainly on the integrity of the cabin to withstand the pressure differential between the ambient and the cabin pressure. Pressurized aircraft are designed to withstand a differential betwen 7.5 and 8.7 psi (pounds per square inch). Safety dictates that the differential level for a particular aircraft is not reached. Excess pressure is therefore vented to the outside.

The pressure differences tolerated by a cabin very much depends on the weakest areas of the cabin walls, which explains why most windows are so small. There are unseen areas that are difficult to seal and where leaks can occur. These are where pipes, wires, and control mechanisms pass through bulkheads. The amount of pressure leak that can be tolerated in maintaining a desired cabin pressure depends on the capacity and efficiency of the compression pumps to replace pressure loss. As mentioned earlier, some leak is intentional. By venting excess cabin pressure to the outside, the differential pressure is kept within safe margins. This also assists in the ventilation of the cabin, so that the same air is not continually being circulated.

Changing Altitude

As there are adverse effects from decreased pressure on certain medical conditions, this might prompt the argument that lower altitudes should be used for aeromedical flights. This is necessarily so in unpressurized aircraft which do not have the choice of flying 20,000 feet or higher. However, there is a choice for pressurized aircraft between flying high where the air is smooth, fuel consumption less, and a faster cruising speed can be maintained, and flying lower where these advantages are absent and where more air turbulence may be experienced.

Flying at lower altitudes eliminates some of the considerations necessary because of decreased pressure, but most of the adverse physiological effects can be compensated for by medical techniques. On balance, it is much more advantageous to fly at higher altitudes in a pressurized plane with regard to the safety and comfort of those on board. Another disadvantage of lower altitudes below 10,000 feet over land and coastal waters is the increased number of other aircraft flying at those levels.

Physiological Effects of
Decreased Atmospheric Pressure

The effects can be divided into those that are related to the *expansion of gases* and those related to the *reduction of available oxygen* (see Oxygenation).

Expansion of Gases.   Two physical laws governing the volume of gases influence the changes that occur with altitude. *Charles' law* states that a given mass of gas under a constant pressure has a volume which is directly proportional to its absolute temperature. *Boyle's law* states that, at constant temperature, the volume of a given mass of gas is inversely proportional to the pressure on it.

How temperature and pressure decrease with altitude has been noted. From the known temperatures and pressures at various altitudes an estimate can be made of the degree of expansion of gases to be expected at particular altitudes (Table 12). The gas-volume expansions are only approximations because of a large number of variables related to local conditions, but they are adequate for the purposes of a medical flight attendant directing the care of a patient.

When *closed or semiclosed body cavities* are considered, a further variable is added. The partial pressure of water vapor, which would normally decrease with altitude, is not decreased as expected because body cavities maintain a saturated level of water vapor through the excretion of moisture from the linings.

When expanding gases are free to maintain equilibrium with the pressure in the cabin as it is changing, there is no danger of excessive positive or negative pressure in an *open cavity* such as the open mouth or unob-

Table 11. Cabin Altitudes from Takeoff to Cruising Altitude.

DC-10[a]		L-1011 Whisperliner[b]	
Minutes from Takeoff	Altitude (feet)	Minutes from Takeoff	Altitude (feet)
0	0	0	0
1	450	1	400
2	1200	2	800
3	1200	3	1100
4	1150	4	1400
5	1050	5	1800
6	950	6	2000
7	750	7	2400
8	575	8	2700
9	800	9	3000
10	1100	10	3000 Level flight
11	1300		
12	1600		
13	2100	27	3100
14	2500	28	3500
15	2850	29	3900
16	3200	30	4500
17	3350	31	5100
18	3500	32	5800
19	3700	33	5900
20	3950	34	6000 Level flight
21	4100		
22	4400		

DC-10: Mean rate of climb, 200 ft/min

L-1011 Whisperliner: Mean rate of climb, 300 ft/min; Mean rate of climb, 400 ft/min

Minutes from Touch Down	Altitude (feet)		Minutes from Touch Down	Altitude (feet)
25	5000		60	6200
24	5000			
23	4800			
18			18	5800
17			17	5400
16			16	5000
15			15	4600
14			14	4300
13			13	4000
12			12	3600
11			11	3300
10	2800		10	2900
9½	2400		9	2500
9	2100		8	2200
8	1800		7	1800
7	1400		6	1400
6	1100		5	1000
5	800		4	800
4	400		3	500
3	100		2	500
2	0		1	200
1	0			

(Cruising altitude 32,000 feet) — Mean rate of descent, 300 ft/min

(Cruising altitude 35,000 feet) — Mean rate of descent, 400 ft/min

[a] American Airlines Flight 653, New York to San Juan, 12/18/81.
[b] Eastern Airlines Flight 920, San Juan to New York, 1/5/82.

Table 12.   Volume Expansion of
Gases.

Altitude (feet)	Altitude (meters)	Gas Volume
0	0	1.0
5,000	1,500	1.2
10,000	3,000	1.5
15,000	4,500	1.9
18,000	5,400	2.0
20,000	6,000	2.4

structed nasopharynx. A *semiclosed cavity* is one with a *restricted outlet* that may or may not allow equalization of pressures, depending on the ease and rapidity with which air can traverse the restriction (e.g., facial sinuses and middle ear).

When a cavity is closed or semiclosed, positive or negative pressure can be harmful and/or painful if equilibrium cannot be achieved with the cabin pressure. This was possibly the first observation made during the infancy of aviation medicine when Charles Roberts reported pain in one ear after the second manned balloon flight in history. He deduced that the pain was due to expansion of air in the inner ear. The flight took place on December 1st, 1783 from Paris and reached the altitude of about 9000 feet. Of course, Benjamin Franklin was there to watch!

The pressure that can build up or act negatively (vacuum effect) in a closed or semiclosed cavity also depends on the resilience of the cavity wall and its ability to expand to accommodate the increased volume or collapse with decreased volume. The facial sinuses, being in bony structures, have little resilience other than the soft tissue comprising the linings. Positive or negative pressure in these cavities can be extremely painful if the ostia fail to allow equalization of pressures. Ostia and ducts have the best chance of remaining patent and functioning adequately when the rate of climb or descent is not too severe. As with eustachian obstruction, relief may be obtained by using a nasal decongestant in a spray form. If pain in the sinuses is debilitating and nasal sprays have not been successful, an aircraft may have to change altitude in the appropriate direction to bring about relief.

Besides the ear and sinus cavities, there are other situations where collections of gas can give rise to problems with altitude.

Gas in the body:
1. Gastrointestinal conditions
2. Pneumothorax
3. Perforating eye injuries
4. Dental cavities
5. Air introduced into cavities during diagnostic procedures
6. Air introduced into tissue during trauma

Gas in equipment:
1. Orthopedic air splints
2. Pneumatic antishock suits
3. Air in intravenous fluid reservoirs
4. Pressure cuffs
5. Balloon cuffs on tracheal and esophageal airways
6. Medication and suction bottles

Problems of Gas Expansion

The medical techniques in dealing with the problems will be covered in sections addressing the physiological changes in the various systems.

GI Tract. There is normally gas in the GI tract, more or less depending on diet, manners of eating, air-swallowing habits, and the ability to eliminate gas upwards or downwards. In healthy individuals, expansion of intestinal gas rarely causes any significant problem because of the resilience of the visceral walls. Cramps and pain can occur when gas is excessive or the abdominal wall is restricted by tight clothing or restraining devices. Sudden expansion of gas in the splenic flexure can trigger a vagal reaction with pain and syncope which can closely mimic the symptoms of a myocardial infarction. Gas expansion in a closed-loop intestinal obstruction can cause a serious deterioration of the condition, and a partial obstruction can be converted into a complete one. A diseased bowel, such as one weakened by ulceration or diverticulitis, may not tolerate an increased pressure and may perforate. The same applies to newly sutured anastomoses. Gaseous distension of the stomach can limit the depression of the diaphragm and compromise respiratory vital capacity. Air, which has obtained entry into the biliary tree through a disease process, can cause fast deterioration of the condition should it expand.

Pneumothorax. Any pneumothorax must be treated prior to medical transfer by air. Even a small pneumothorax will expand at altitude and in doing so may tear healing adhesions causing bleeding or become a tension pneumothorax. When a patient is transported by air with a chest tube in place, the tube must not be closed and a valve is necessary.

The importance of pneumothorax in the aviation environment might be judged from the fact that most air forces exclude men from flight training if they have a history of spontaneous pneumothorax. Should a spontaneous pneumothorax occur in a fully trained pilot, he will be grounded until surgery is performed to seal the intrapleural space. He will not be allowed to resume flying duties until an attempt to produce an artificial pneumothorax is shown to fail.

The Injured Eye. An injured eye is very susceptible to hypoxia and to pressure changes. Extrusion of global contents can occur when the atmospheric pressure decreases in the cabin.

Dental Cavities. Modern dental techniques usually assure that air is not trapped when a cavity is filled. An apical abscess can form gases according to the nature of the infection. Expansion of this gas is extremely limited by the structures of the alveolar socket, and the resultant increase in pressure can cause severe pain.

Air from Diagnostic Procedures. The introduction of air into cavities for radiological reasons, such as for an air encephalogram, presents a serious hazard for an air transfer patient. Sufficient time must elapse after such a procedure for the air to be absorbed before a flight can be made. Air introduced into a joint at the time of arthroscopy can cause severe pain if it is allowed to expand.

Trauma. When an open wound has been treated, there may be some air trapped in it. Irrigation of wounds (much to be commended) occasionally drives air into tissue planes, and all of the air may not escape as the irrigation fluid drains. The expansion of air in soft tissue may not cause a problem, but it could feasibly exert extra tension on suture lines or locally compress the capillary circulation. It becomes a much greater importance when a limb is rigidly enclosed in a plaster cast. In such cases, even a small amount of swelling provoked by expansion of air can set the stage for circulatory embarrassment.

Air Expansion in Equipment

Orthopedic Air Splints and Pneumatic Antishock Suits. It can be deduced what hazards may present themselves should the air expand in an air splint applied to a limb or in a pneumatic suit such as the military antishock trousers (MAST pants). Careful monitoring of the pressures in them can prevent harm and maintain their usefulness.

Air in Intravenous Reservoirs. How flow is regulated in an environment where pressures are changing is addressed elsewhere, but note should be made at this time of a certain danger. Inflatable cuffs are sometimes necessary to increase the pressure above a reservoir and maintain a reasonable flow. The added pressure with expansion of the air within the cuff could cause an air embolus under the right circumstances. This also applies to cuffs around pliable, collapsible reservoirs.

When rigid glass bottles must be used as the reservoir, the air inlet may require pressure to be pumped into it by manual means. In this case, the air above the fluid may be subject to expansive forces that are prevented from venting. This can also cause air embolus.

Pressure Cuffs. Blood pressure cuffs might be only partially deflated between measurements and may tighten without a complaint from an unconscious patient. This might not be noticed until the next time a blood pressure reading was attempted.

Balloon Cuffs. The balloon cuffs on some endotracheal tubes and esophageal airways may contain air pressures that can put undue strain on the lining of the trachea or esophagus should no compensation be made for gas expansion by adjustment on change of altitude.

Bottles. The problem with screw-cap medicine and suction bottles is how tightly to turn the lids to make sure they don't leak and how loosely to adjust them so that they do not become unopenable because of pressures on the screw threads. This problem can be partly solved by ensuring the absolute cleanliness of the cap and rim and by lubrication with a minute amount of vaseline. Snap-capped vials will occasionally pop open, mixing hard-to-identify pills.

Warning from the Laundry
The most universally used instrument in the practice of medicine is the ballpoint pen. The design of some pens causes shirts and uniforms to be ruined. Ink may discharge should a tiny vent hole become blocked and cabin pressures fall. Fountain pens are even worse, but are not often to be found in aircraft these days. There are no problems with gas expansion when using a pencil.

Sudden Decompression
The effects of gaseous expansion, compression, and reduction (previously mentioned) are mainly concerned with the rates of pressure change to be found on aeromedical flights. Accidents do happen and sudden decompression can occur. This could be due to structural defects (especially in windows and doors), to violence occurring in the cabin, or to the integrity of the fuselage being disrupted by a missile from the outside. When decompression occurs suddenly, the effects of pressure change previously described are exaggerated, the alveolar sacs of the lungs act as semiclosed cavities, hypoxia is an immediate danger, and cabin temperatures drop dramatically. (See Emergencies in the Air later in this Part for details of how to survive such a disaster.)

OXYGENATION

The aviation environment adds a number of factors to oxgyen therapy that are usually absent in a hospital setting.

Sources of Oxygen

Most of the oxygen used in hospitals is stored as a gas in cylinders. In aviation, there are four sources of supply that are alternatively used: GOX, LOX, SOX, and OBOGS.

1. GOX—oxygen as a gas under pressure
2. LOX—liquid oxygen
3. SOX—oxygen generated from solid chemicals
4. OBOGS (on board oxygen generating system)—oxygen generated from ambient air

GOX
The best known and the most commonly used method of carrying oxygen is in an elongated cylinder into which gaseous oxygen has been compressed. The advantages of this method are: relative simplicity of the systems involved, some assurance of purity at the point of use, less-complicated maintenance, a reasonable amount can be stored, and it can be replenished at many airports around the world. Its main disadvantage

Table 13. Capacities of Oxygen Cylinders.

Cylinder Size	Capacity (liters) at 70°F, 14.7 psi	Cylinder Weight (Full) (lbs)
D	356	11
E	622	16
G	1200	32
Q	2320	70
H and K	6900	150

in aviation is the weight of the cylinders when a small-payload light aircraft is used.

Those companies that produce oxygen for sale and distribution often produce three grades of oxygen: commercial, medical, and aviation. The commercial variety may not have a standard of purity for medical use and is mainly used for welding. There is some misunderstanding of the difference between medical and aviation oxygen. Both have a regulated degree of purity, and the main difference is the allowable level of humidity accepted. Aviation oxygen must not contain more than 0.005 mg of water per liter of oxygen measured at 15°C and 760 mm Hg. Medical oxygen may contain more than this amount and is often purposely humidified.

In some countries, different authorities regulate the degree of purity of aviation and medical oxgyen. An aviation authority may specify the required purity of oxygen to be used on aircraft. A health authority may publish a pharmacopoeia establishing purity levels. In general, all authorities specify similar standards with regard to certain aspects of purity.

If oxygen is to be used by man, it must be at least 99.5% oxygen when it is supplied as a gas. It must be free from odor and not contain any toxic substances. If carbon monoxide is present, it must be less than 0.002%.

Oxygen cylinders used on board aircraft must be able to tolerate internal pressures of 1800 psi. Most of the cylinders are made of steel (the type and strength also regulated). Some are made of other alloys which are lighter, but they must still meet certain specifications for pressure tolerance. Table 13 gives some indication of the capacity of the average steel oxygen cylinder that will be used in the United States and what its weight might be when full. The cylinder-size coding is that commonly used for medical oxygen in the U.S.

All oxygen cylinders taken on board at the commencement of an air medical transfer mission *must* be filled to the maximum registered capacity. The responsibility for this should be shared by the medical flight attendant and the pilot in command. The pilot will also be responsible that all other oxygen cylinders which are incorporated into the regular equipment of the aircraft for use by the crew and passengers (as per F.A.R., Part 23) are filled to capacity.

LOX

Oxygen can be stored in a liquid form. The system to do so is more complicated than the simple storage of the gas under pressure in cylinders. It is mainly used in military aircraft in which more consideration has to be given to the space a system will occupy and how much it will weigh. While it is currently being used as a portable system for aeromedical use, it is perhaps only appropriate for short-range missions after which the aircraft returns to its base where the LOX unit can be replenished.

At many airports, the facility to recharge the unit will not be present. The unit has to be charged immediately before a mission because there is a leakage that starts to occur approximately 10 hours after recharging. From that point, leakage continues at an approximate rate of 10% in 24 hours.

The main advantage of the system is its lighter weight and smaller volume, but there are other disadvantages besides leakage. There is a greater chance that the patient might receive contaminated oxygen and, therefore, complicated testing of the unit must be performed at regular intervals. Any contaminants that could enter the system are condensed at each recycling and could eventually reach toxic levels by forming a concentrated particle that would evaporate in the warming coils and suddenly give a high concentration on inhalation. Also note that LOX is more expensive than GOX.

SOX

Oxygen can be generated by adding heat (through some controllable trigger mechanism) to a matrix of sodium chlorate and iron powder; these chemicals are stored as solid candles. However, this reaction is not free from the formation of contaminants including carbon monoxide and free chlorine. Adding barium peroxide to the materials in the candle neutralizes these impurities, so that the oxygen generated for medical use is within the limits for purity required by the various regulating authorities. It is 99.9% pure without toxic contaminants.

Once a generator has been triggered to produce oxygen, it continues to do so until the unit is exhausted. It cannot be turned on and off as required. Each unit will produce oxygen at a specific rate (decided by the design of the candle) for a specific length of time. The time of production is not very long. Depending on the unit or the number of units triggered together, 10 to 40 minutes of oxygen supply can be expected.

The above information explains why SOX is not suitable for medical use where flow rates may need to be changed or stopped and long periods of use might be needed. It is used in some aircraft as the emergency supply of oxygen for the crew and passengers should pressurization fail. Portable units are sometimes carried so that crew members can move about the aircraft and perform duties during a period when supplementary oxygen is essential. It is useful in this respect and can provide a short-term backup supply for a patient should other systems fail or be depleted.

The author has found portable SOX units to have another disadvantage. Spare candles can be stored to recharge the unit so that it will work again. This entails removing the depleted candle, which is very hot just after burnout, with a metal device. It is not too difficult to burn one's hand while removing the core, and the chance of this happening increases manyfold if it has to be done in an aircraft in turbulent air.

One of the more useful models of portable oxygen supply is named the AVIOX DUO-PAK, made by Scott Aviation (Fig. 26). It is basically

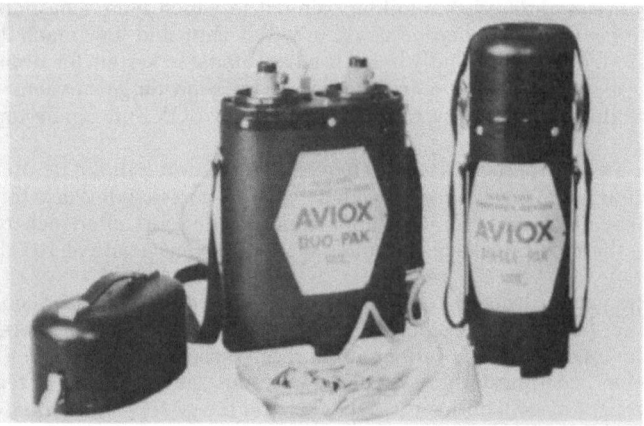

Figure 26. Solid oxygen system (Aviox). (Courtesy of Scott Aviation, Lancaster, New York.)

twin single units that can be discharged singly or together. Singly, the unit provides 4 liters per minute of oxygen for 40 minutes. If both cores are triggered simultaneously, an instant flow at 8 liters per minute will continue for 20 minutes. The weight of the unit with the assembly cover, mask and tubing, and generator cores in place is 8.25 lbs. The generator cores can be stored for a considerable amount of time without deterioration. This type of SOX equipment could be useful as a backup system for supplemental oxygen and could find use at the pickup point of a mission when portable oxygen is not available for the transport of the patient from the dispatching hospital or location of the patient to the airfield.

OBOGS

There have been a number of systems developed to generate oxygen on board an aircraft other than the SOX method. Most have proved impractical for one reason or another. However, a method that has found some acceptance is one which depends on molecular sieves and has been named OBOGS, developed by the Bendix Corporation. OBOGS requires electrical power for the concentrator and the oxygen monitor. The concentrator uses bleed air from the engines and alternately passes it through two molecular sieves which remove the nitrogen which is then vented. The inlet air must be heated and filtered before entering the sieves. The oxygen monitor uses a polarographic oxygen sensor to continuously measure the partial pressure of oxygen in the produced gas. It signals any fall below a predetermined level and turns on a reserve of gaseous oxygen. The most up-to-date models have been made capable of producing a 95% concentration of oxygen. They are reputed to be reliable to the extent that some have been tested over 4000 hours before failure.

The place of OBOGS in aeromedical care has yet to be determined. It has no weight advantage over the LOX system. It is possible that its use could be considered when ambulance aircraft are extremely active and operating in regions where GOX, LOX, and SOX supplies are sparse or unreliable.

Economy of Use

Unlimited amounts of oxygen cannot be carried on each mission. In some cases, not much in excess of the estimated needs can be carried. Should the oxygen supply become exhausted in flight, the medical flight attendant cannot telephone the supply department of the hospital to deliver another cylinder immediately. Special care must therefore be taken to economize on oxygen use by ensuring there is no avoidable waste of the gas. The prevention of leaks in equipment, connections, adapters, and hoses also acts as a safety measure. The choice of face mask for the patient, how well it seals, and using the minimum flow that will provide satisfactory oxygenation can conserve oxygen. Cracking an oxygen cylinder (initial opening to start flow from the high pressure in the cylinder through the reducing valve) before connecting the low-pressure flow line to the patient does waste some oxygen but is an essential safety measure.

Estimation of Amount Required

The amount of oxygen that might be required should be estimated in advance. The estimation must take into account possible changes in the flight time, whether replenishment will be possible at the turnround point, and must allow an adequate reserve for emergency use. Table 14 gives an indication of how long various sizes of cylinders will provide oxygen at particular flow rates. The usable capacity is empirically calculated, making allowances for unavoidable loss such as from cracking the cylinder and for the variable factors such as temperature changes and inaccuracies in flow measurements. The cylinder-size coding is the same as in Table 13.

Methods of Delivery

Retrofitted Oxygen Supply Systems

In those aircraft which have a built-in oxygen system, the reservoir cylinders can be topped up to their maximum capacity of 1800 psi from larger cylinders on trolleys outside the aircraft. The larger cylinders have a maximum pressure of 3600 psi. In order that the reservoir system be protected from pressures it cannot tolerate, reducing valves are necessary in stages. Similarly, the low-pressure lines which carry the oxygen to the positions of use (outlets at crew stations and in the cabin) are protected from the high cylinder pressures by reducing valves. The flow at the outlets is automatically determined by the altitude at which the aircraft is flying (in unpressurized aircraft). This is done by having a regulator in line which is sensitive to the in-plane atmospheric pressure through an aneroid sensor. In the U.S., each system is rated to provide sufficient oxygen for normal operations up to a specified altitude when it meets the requirements of F.A.R. Part 23, 1443.

All systems do not have an altitude-compensated regulator, especially

Table 14. Estimated Endurance of O_2 Supply (in hours/minutes) Related to Flow Rate when Used in Air Transport.

Cylinder Size	Usable Capacity (liters)	Flow Rates (liters/min)				
		2	4	6	8	10
D	300	2h 30m	1h 15m	50m	35m	30m
E	600	5h	2h 30m	1h 40m	1h 10m	1h
G	1000	8h 20m	4h 10m	2h 45m	2h 5m	1h 40m
Q	2000	16h 40m	8h 20m	5h 30m	4h 10m	3h 20m
H and K	6500	54h	27h	18h	13h 30m	11h

in small aircraft, and manual control is necessary. All systems can be initiated or turned off manually. These constant-flow systems are designed primarily to enable unpressurized aircraft to fly over 10,000 feet, at which level supplementary oxygen becomes necessary for relatively normal, healthy individuals. It is suitable for patients who have no increased susceptibility to hypoxia. The ill or injured patient often has a need for more oxygen than these systems provide. Therefore, other sources of oxygen must be carried. Oxygen systems designed to provide emergency oxygen on sudden decompression of a pressurized aircraft will be described later.

There are gauges in the cockpit to inform the pilot of the state of readiness of built-in oxygen systems. Some aircraft have an indicator on the outside skin of the plane which can be inspected on a walkaround check. It shows a green disk if there is no leak in the system; the disk snaps out if there is a leak. The device is made by Scott Aviation Products, who manufacture many of the aircraft oxygen systems.

For a patient who has a specific range to his oxygen requirements, it is important that the medical flight attendant know the flow rate of any oxygen being supplied as well as the approximate percentage of oxygen being supplied to the patient's respiratory tract. The flow rate also needs to be known to have some idea of how long a supply will last. Not all flowmeters are accurate in the aviation environment.

Modifications of Equipment

The flowmeter most commonly used to measure the flow of oxygen being delivered to a patient in the hospital is the Thorpe tube flowmeter. It is the one with a floating ball in a tube. These flowmeters are not all compensated for back pressure. Those that are not are affected by a reduction in the atmospheric pressure as occurs at altitude. For them to be compensated so that the readings maintain some accuracy, the needle valve must be downstream to the tube. Inertial forces acting on the ball with climb, descent, acceleration, and deceleration can affect the accuracy, especially if the tube is not vertical to the axis of the cabin. They can be used for aeromedical work if they are compensated for back pressure, are kept vertical, and accuracy of flow rates is not imperative.

Flowmeters which are an integral part of regulator valves are affected to some extent by altitude. Inaccuracies only begin when flow rates in excess of 6 liters per minute are used over 5000 feet. These inaccuracies do not have too much significance below 8000 feet. One of the more reliable oxygen-metering devices is the Robertshaw constant flow selector valve, manufactured by the Robertshaw Control Company (Fig. 27).

Other modifications of oxygenation equipment concern themselves with EMI output, operational voltages, and independent battery supply of power. Excess EMI (electromagnetic interference) can interfere with an aircraft's navigational instruments. Electrically powered respirators and suction equipment should be chosen that are adequately shielded and produce minimum EMI. All electrically powered apparatus to be used for aeromedical missions should have an internal battery supply of power. Retrofitted outlets may have varying voltages, and power may not be available from the outlets on engine shutdown.

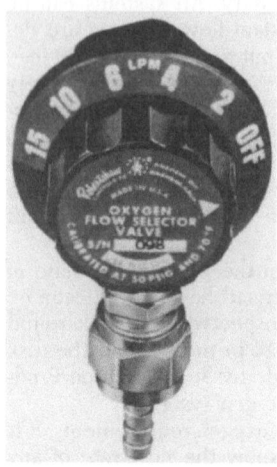

Figure 27. Constant flow selector valve. This unit is also available with flow settings of 1, 2, 3, 4, and 8 liters per minute as well as an off position. (Courtesy of Robertshaw Control Company, Anaheim, California.)

Hypoxia

Except for emergency situations of decompression of the cabin, patients traveling in pressurized aircraft will not have to tolerate a cabin altitude of more than 8000 feet. Some unpressurized flights may have to climb above 8000 feet to traverse mountainous areas. For this reason, the effects of diminished oxygen tension in the atmosphere up to 15,000 feet must be addressed.

A patient who has suffered a pulmonary embolus might well have a Pa_{O_2} of less than 60 mm Hg on room air. This is the same Pa_{O_2} to be expected in a healthy adult at approximately 6000 feet, conditions of temperature, humidity, metabolism, and respiratory functions being constant. It could be considered that this patient with the pulmonary embolus has an oxygenation status while on the ground equivalent to 6000 feet. The same patient may require supplementary oxygenation at 6000 feet, equivalent to what would be required by a physiologically intact person at 12,000 feet.

The carbon monoxide inhaled by cigarette smokers reduces the available oxyhemoglobin to the extent that a smoker can be considered to be at an altitude of 2000 feet when at sea level. This may be the origin of the term "high" when related to smoking and ingesting drugs.

When preparing to transfer a patient by air, it is convenient to be able to judge his condition with a view to determining his *altitude-equivalent* with regard to his oxygenation status. Two other variables must also be taken into account when making this estimate:

1. Estimate is made from judgments of the medical condition while the patient is being provided some artificial assistance to improve the oxygenation status *or* while the patient is *not* being given any assistance.
2. The height of the patient above sea level at the time the estimate is being made. (How long the patient has been at that height and from

what altitude levels was the patient moved before the estimate can sometimes be significant.)

If the hypoxic effects of altitude to be considered are those in healthy adults and those altitudes refer to the number of feet above *sea level*, a rough estimate of the oxygenation requirements of a patient may be assisted by using an altitude-equivalent value.

The Patient's Equivalent Altitude

$$SLEAC = NA - LA + RTA$$

where SLEAC is a resting patient's equivalent altitude above sea level (sea level equivalent altitude compensated); NA is that altitude at which a healthy adult would exhibit the same oxygenation deficiencies exhibited by the patient at the height the estimate is being made; LA is the altitude of the location of the patient above sea level; and RTA is that altitude equivalent represented by the oxygenation being provided the patient (respiratory therapy) as it would relate to the supplementary oxygen requirements of a healthy adult to maintain adequate oxygenation of the tissues at that altitude.

Oxygenation refers to that of the blood and tissues and not to that available to the respiratory tract. All the oxygen in the world available to the respiratory tract will not provide adequate oxygenation of the tissues if the circulating volume of blood is insufficient or there are not enough red blood cells with an adequate hemoglobin content in that circulation. How various medical conditions affect the efficiency of oxygenation of the tissues and examples of SLEAC estimates are given later. First, an understanding of the effects of altitude and its associated hypoxia on healthy adults is essential.

Hypoxia Increased with Altitude

As was apparent in the study of the atmosphere, the atmospheric pressure decreases with altitude. With this decrease in pressure, the volume of a given mass of air increases proportionately. The pressure exerted by each gas in the air is reduced at the same rate as the total atmospheric pressure because the composition of air remains constant at the heights with which we are concerned.

We know the atmospheric pressure of air falls from 760 mm Hg at sea level to 380 mm Hg at 18,000 feet. The partial pressure of oxygen at sea level is 159 mm Hg (21% of 760 mm Hg). At 18,000 feet, the partial pressure of oxygen is only 80 mm Hg in the air available for respiration. That this is a meager supply of oxygen is realized when the relationship between atmospheric P_{O_2} and an expected arterial $P_{O_2}(Pa_{O_2})$ is known (Table 15).

Although it is interesting to know the oxygen tension in the inspired air, it is the oxygen tension in the alveoli which determines the availability of oxygen to the vasculopulmonary system. The oxygen tension in the alveolar gas is not the same as in the inspired gas because of the carbon dioxide tension in the alveoli. The CO_2 tension remains relatively constant between sea level and 8000 feet if the ratio of carbon dioxide expired to alveolar ventilation does not change.

Table 15. Altitude, Atmospheric Pressure, and Blood Gases.

Altitude			
Feet	Meters	Atmospheric P_{O_2}	Arterial P_{O_2}
Sea Level		159	98
2000	600	148	86
4000	1200	137	73
6000	1800	125	64
8000	2400	116	55

The alveolar oxygen tension decreases with altitude in a linear manner up to 8000 feet in an individual not having any abnormality that would limit oxygen uptake or alter carbon dioxide production and who maintains a normal physiologically regulated ventilatory rate and capacity (Fig. 28). The linear nature of the decrease with altitude does not continue above 8000 feet. Above 8000 feet, the Pa_{O_2} falls to a level which stimulates increased ventilation, reducing alveolar CO_2 tension. Because of this, there is a relative rise in the alveolar oxygen tension, and the tension does not fall as steeply with further increase in altitude.

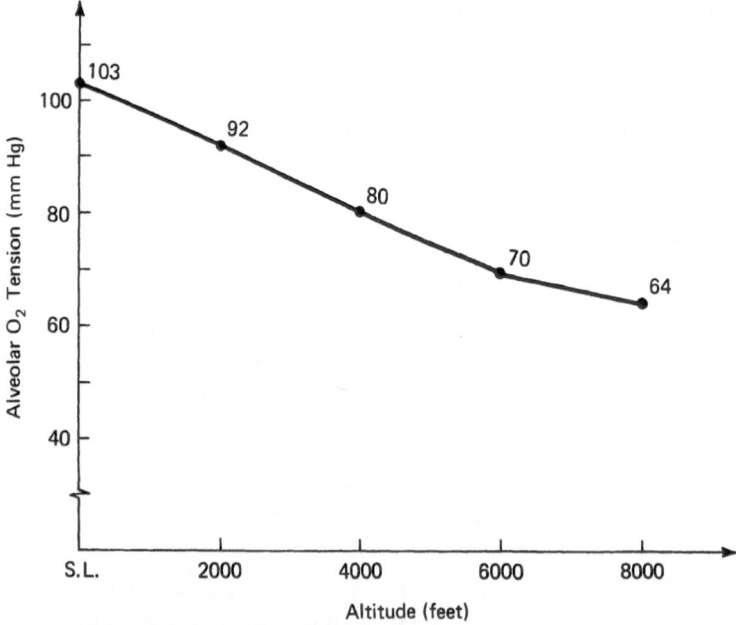

Figure 28. Alveolar oxygen tension related to altitude.

Table 16.   Physiologic Effects of Altitude Secondary to Hypoxia.

Sea level to 4000 ft (O_2 saturation more than 93%)
No Hypoxic symptoms.

4000–5000 ft (O_2 saturation below 95%)
Diminished night vision. (The retina is sensitive to small levels of hypoxia.) A resting subject performing minor mental tasks might show no change in performance, but the ability to perform novel mental tasks may be impaired.

5000–8000 ft (O_2 saturation below 92%)
Ability to perform skilled tasks impaired. Capacity to perform physical work reduced. Fatigue has earlier onset.

8000–10,000 ft (O_2 saturation below 90%)
Mental and physical abilities reduced. Day vision may be impaired. Headaches and noticeable fatigue can occur.

10,000–14,000 ft (O_2 saturation below 85%)
Handicaps would become increasingly apparent if the degree of euphoria that can accompany the handicaps did not mask them from the subject. Some subjects are aware of the handicaps which are: loss of critical judgment, unreliability of mental calculations, ability to concentrate on particular tasks diminished with either unnecessarily prolonged attention to the task or diminished attention span. More severe fatigue.

14,000–16,000 ft (O_2 saturation below 80%)
Neuromuscular control deteriorates. Psychomotor performance unreliable. Slow thought processing. Emotional states may surface related to basic personality traits of a similar nature as those exhibited with alcoholic intoxication. Lightheadedness. More severe headaches. Paresthesias may be suffered, hindering touch and grasp sensation. Increase in the rate and depth of ventilation. Physical exertion may provoke syncope.

16,000–18,000 ft (O_2 saturation below 72%)
Severe handicaps. Unable to perform flying duties or attend to others. Physical effort leads to coma.

18,000–20,000 ft (O_2 saturation below 70%)
Unconsciousness occurs with minimal warning but sometimes preceded by anoxic convulsions. Death will ensue if oxygen support is not provided or if the aircraft does not return to lower altitudes.

Up to approximately 18,000 feet, there is some balance between the *stimulation of ventilation* by the falling oxygen tension acting through the carotid and aortic chemoreceptors and the *inhibition of ventilation* produced through the falling CO_2 tension acting on central sensors. The balance is not achieved concomitantly with the oxygen and carbon dioxide tension changes but takes some time to reach the point where the acid-base balance is effective and relatively stable. This balanced situation does not continue for very long before the physiologic compensatory mechanisms are exhausted unless there has been a slow acclimatization over days or weeks. This acclimatization is applicable to sensible mountain climbers but not to aeromedical missions, except in exceptional circumstances.

Even before compensatory increase in ventilation comes into play, the reduced oxygen tension of altitude produces symptoms. The early symptoms may be mild, or they may be missing if the rate of ascent is severe, bringing about more serious symptoms which may be very acute and disastrous in an aviator unprotected by supplementary oxygen. Table 16 describes the symptoms in relation to altitude levels and the corresponding oxygen saturation levels common at those altitudes. It should be obvious from the table that no patient, crew member, medical attendant, or any other person on board should be exposed to cabin altitudes of more than 10,000 feet without supplemental oxygen. A patient with some degree of hypoxia at sea level or with a condition that predisposes to minor degrees of hypoxia must have supplemental oxygen at the lower altitudes below 8000 feet. These are the altitudes which might be experienced in the cabin of a pressurized aircraft.

It must be repeated that the subject of the present discussion is a healthy adult and *not* an ill or injured patient. Neither is the subject a smoker nor has he imbibed alcohol during the previous 8 hours. He is relatively calm, cool, and collected and occupies an aircraft cabin with a comfortable temperature and that is not subject to any significant turbulence. He is not acclimatized to altitude, and his exposure is that to be expected in normal civilian aviation should he break regulations and continue above 10,000 feet without supplemental oxygen in an unpressurized cabin.

Acclimatization

It was pointed out that the effects of altitude described would be those experienced by unacclimatized individuals. Many people live at altitudes above 10,000 feet. The physiological compensations that allow them to tolerate higher altitudes have been achieved more gradually than is possible in flight.

It is interesting to note that the nurses flying missions with the Flying Doctors of Africa report minimal problems flying at 15,000 feet without supplementary oxygen. Their base, Wilson Airport in Nairobi, is 6000 feet above sea level. If they were based in Mombassa or Malindi on the coast, effects would have been more apparent. It is possible that effects at 15,000 feet went unnoticed because of the nature of the symptoms that can occur.

The Hypoxic Patient at Ground Level

Not all hospitals around the world can offer blood gas measurements. In those that can, the Pa_{O_2} of a patient who is at rest breathing room air without hyperventilating can be related to the expected Pa_{O_2} of our healthy aviator at various altitudes. This would provide the altitude equivalent (NA) (Fig. 29). Estimating the NA and knowing the height of the hospital (LA) will allow you to calculate the patient's SLEAC (com-

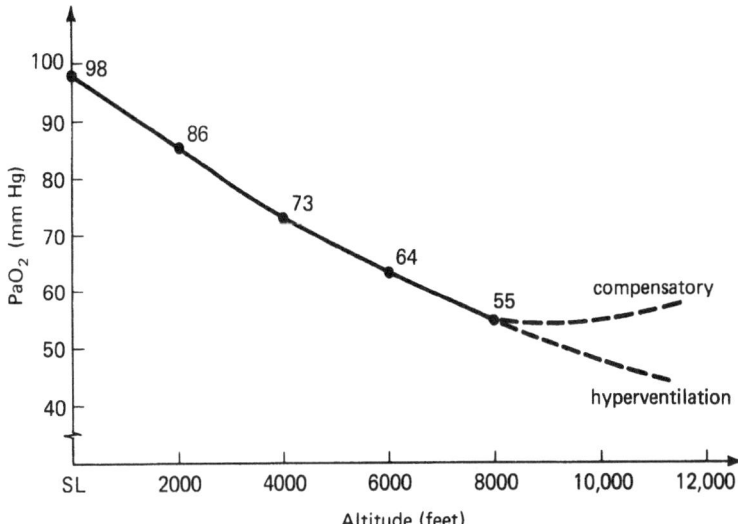

Figure 29. Expected Pa$_{O_2}$ of healthy adults at various altitudes. The altitude equivalent (NA) of a hypoxic patient can be determined if the Pa$_{O_2}$ in room air is known.

pensated equivalent altitude). Should the patient be in a location where arterial blood gases are not available, clinical acumen must be relied upon.

Two methods can be tried to estimate the altitude equivalent of a hypoxic patient. The first involves judging cerebral function and relating it to the changes which occur in our healthy aviator at altitude. This will not take into account cerebral deficiencies the patient may have due to age, disease, or toxicity. The second involves a diagnostic oxygen challenge. Physical examination of the patient with regard to skin and mucous membranes, pulse and blood pressure, peripheral circulation, urine (character and output), degree of dyspnea, and cerebral acuity should give some indication of the degree of hypoxia present. If oxygen is provided in increasing concentrations at a constant flow rate of 4 liters per minute until the majority of the signs which indicated hypoxia have subsided, the minimum percentage of oxygen required can be related to the range of altitude where that percentage of oxygen is necessary to compensate for hypoxia.

The point of estimating the patient's SLEAC is to have some idea of the degree of supplementary oxygenation he will require at those altitudes to be experienced. Whether positive pressure equipment will be needed should become obvious. Patients requiring 40% or more of oxygen at ground level will need respirators on missions to be flown over 4000 feet. Patients already on positive pressure respirators at ground level will always need a respirator in flight at any altitude.

Influences on FiO_2 Requirements

Conditions requiring increased FiO_2.

1. Increased metabolic rate: longer term—thyrotoxicosis; current—increased body temperature, high (and very low) environmental temperatures (on the ground and in the cabin).
2. Decreased effective circulating volume.
3. Anemia.
4. Thoracic or airway injury (however minor).

Conditions requiring a decrease in FiO_2:[3]

1. Polycythemia rubra vera with compensated cardiovascular status.
2. Compensatory polycythemia associated with chronic obstructive pulmonary disease.
3. Chronic emphysema with persistent hypercapnia.
4. Neurotic patients known to frequently hyperventilate during anxious episodes. The symptoms of respiratory alkalosis can have an earlier onset at altitudes where there has already been a reduction in the alveolar CO_2 from the degree of compensatory hyperventilation. This is most likely to occur above 8000 feet.

If the FiO_2 that is adequate for the patient's oxygen needs at ground level is known, a table can be used to estimate the FiO_2 that will be necessary at various altitudes to give an equivalent level of oxygenation (Table 17).

Steep Hypoxic Gradient

Review of *hypoxia with altitude* in many aviation medicine texts, texts on respiratory physiology in general medicine, and pulmonary medicine textbooks provides paradoxical information. Since most of these texts show striking similarities, one must conclude that many are reviews of some original text. Unfortunately, the original text presented some confusing information that has been passed on in succeeding texts. As far as the author is aware, no text is available that satisfactorily clarifies the paradox.

All the texts describe the oxygen dissociation curve and its modification by various factors such as CO_2 levels, pH, and temperature. How the oxygen-hemoglobin buffer system maintains oxygen tension at the cellular level is then explained. However, information is generally missing which would modify the conclusions to be drawn, although clues are provided in chapters on cellular metabolism. Without the missing information, the apparent conclusion is that the human body has a system adaptable to hypoxia and that this system maintains adequate oxygenation levels for individual cells.

The paradox appears when the same texts go on to describe the symptoms of altitude related to the increasing hypoxia. The first symptoms appear around 5000 to 6000 feet. The adaptation system must therefore be quickly overcome in the aviation environment or have some serious

---

[3] Patients with conditions 1–3 may be sensitive to any reduction of Pa_{CO_2}, and the hypoventilation that might occur will not be compensated for by the hyperventilatory stimulation from a low Pa_{O_2} if FiO_2 is too high.

Table 17. Percent of Oxygen Concentrations Required to Maintain a Pa_{O_2} of 100 mm Hg.

Meters	0	400	1200	1800	2400	3000
Feet	0	2000	4000	6000	8000	10,000
	21	23	25	27	29	32
	30	33	35	38	42	45
	40	44	47	51	55	60
	50	54	59	64	69	75
FiO_2	60	65	70	76	83	90
	70	76	82	90	97	100
	80	87	94	100	/////	/////
	90	98	100	positive pressure required		
	100	100		/////	/////	/////

Note: Preflight assessment Pa_{O_2} values have little use unless the oxygen concentration being provided the patient before the test is reported. Pa_{O_2} and other blood gas measurements must always be associated with a clinical picture to have any value.

defects. Slow adaptation (acclimatization) is more easily understood. An attempt will therefore be made to show why a steep hypoxic gradient (that experienced with the rate of climb in flight) does present a physiological challenge that cannot be totally buffered except by artificial means (supplemental oxygen).

The Oxygen-Hemoglobin Buffer System

The human body has many ways of compensating for deleterious effects on normal physiology. The best known is possibly the acid-base buffer system which maintains a desirable pH in the blood. To tolerate changes in available oxygen at the alveoli and the loss of oxygen tension with reduced blood flow to distant cells, a mechanism is provided whereby a reduced alveolar oxygen tension does not affect the oxygen tension provided to tissue cells to the extent expected. As oxygen tension in the blood reduces, oxygen dissociates from the hemoglobin more easily. Dissociation rates vary at different tensions. At tensions below 70 mm Hg, at which normal blood is about 90% saturated with oxygen, oxygen is released at increasingly faster rates as the oxygen tension decreases (see the steep part of the oxygen dissociation curve in Fig. 30).

There would appear to be an attempt to ensure that the tissues do not

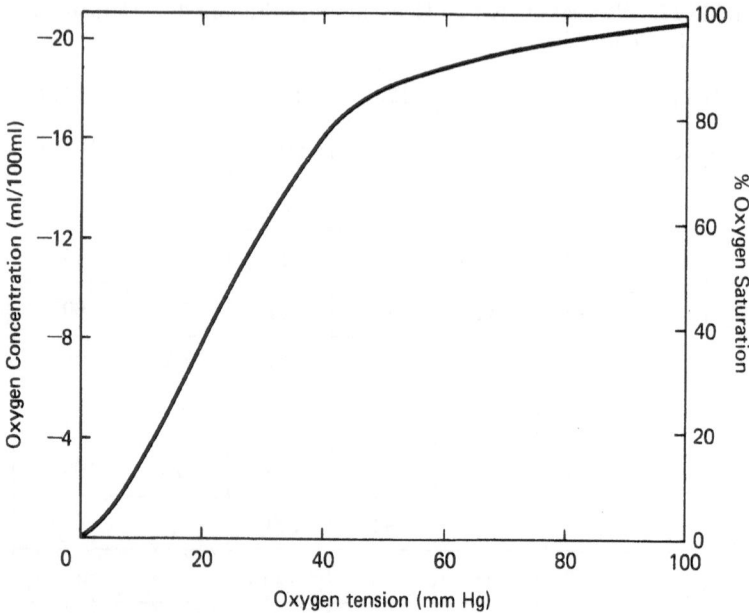

Figure 30. Normal oxygen dissociation curve (15 g of hemoglobin per 100 ml of blood).

suffer hypoxia when the oxygen available to the alveoli is reduced. The system attempts to maintain the oxygen tension available to the tissues at between 20 and 40 mm Hg. A tissue cell is supposed to be able to survive with only 3 to 5 mm Hg oxygen tension. This gives the impression that hypoxia should be tolerated quite well. In fact, the body does not tolerate hypoxia very well at all. A number of factors help to explain why it does not.

Limits of the Oxygen-Hemoglobin Buffer System. Hemoglobin's decreased affinity for oxygen at lower oxygen tensions, which allows the release of larger amounts of oxygen, is also present at the point of oxygen pickup at the alveolar pulmonary membrane. With less affinity for oxygen, less oxygen is picked up when the oxygen tension in the alveoli decreases. At the lower altitudes, a normal subject has sufficient oxygen tension in the alveoli to not reach the steep part of the dissociation curve. However, a patient who has a SLEAC of 4000 or 5000 feet would quickly be on the steep slide without supplemental oxygen.

Oxygen Requirements of Tissue Cells. The figures most often quoted for the buffered oxygen tensions at the tissue level related to alveolar tensi n are those for the total mass of body tissue. It is as though the body is considered one big cell or that all the cells are similar, have the same oxygen requirements, and are provided with the same opportunity of oxygenation with a standard circulatory flow. A cell may survive on an oxygen tension of 3 to 5 mm Hg, but it may not function normally and the physiology may change dramatically within the cell. The point is that cells are far from being all alike, and their oxygen requirements may vary considerably from other cells and within their own group with regard to the varying demands being placed on them at any particular moment.

Protective Circulatory Shifts.   The vascular system, under the influence of the autonomic nervous system and of changes in blood chemistry and levels of endocrine secretions, has the ability to shunt blood supply so that vital organs are given priority. The brain and heart are privileged. The lungs do not have to fight for their share, but the kidneys do to an extent. The adrenal glands (the subphrenic brain) have aortic, phrenic, and renal arteries providing circulation and benefit from priorities placed elsewhere.

Distant Cellular Malfunction Affecting Cells Enjoying More Oxygen.   An unidentified tissue cell may survive with an oxygen tension of only 3 to 5 mm Hg. This does not necessarily mean it survives in a healthy state or functions normally. In general, a cell which is not receiving the optimum amount of oxygen to function at its required level of efficiency has some disorder in its complex biochemical metabolism and excretes unwanted metabolites into the blood. If the underprivileged cell rejects unusual metabolites, it is unlikely that the cells struggling for privilege will welcome those metabolites in the fluids carrying their own nutrition. There is every chance those metabolites will be harmful. An analogy may be drawn from the various effects of better-known metabolites that take their toll in ketosis. One might hypothesize that the detrimental products of hypoxia on distant cells (low-priority users of oxygen) disturb the function of the cells which have been given the priority for oxygenation through protective circulatory shifts.

Hypoxic Effects Not Due to Local Hypoxia.   It is possible that what we term hypoxic symptoms of the brain are in fact not due to oxygen deprivation in the brain itself but rather to the toxic metabolites from hypoxic tissues elsewhere in the body. An experiment that might support this hypothesis involves the investigation of brain death in dogs after cardiac arrest. It was determined that brain death occurred in dogs 4 to 6 minutes after cardiac arrest. The time of brain death after cardiac arrest was then determined after removing all the blood from the brain at the time of arrest. Those brains survived for more then 30 minutes! This would seem to indicate that the products of cellular hypoxia in the blood hasten brain death and that brain death is not simply due to a lack of oxygen.

Conclusion.   The preceding theories offer some explanations of why symptoms occur with the hypoxia associated with altitude. Presenting information on oxygen dissociation and the oxygen-hemoglobin buffer system without further explanation is confusing and may promote questionable decisions by those who care for patients at altitude. This is especially important when the patient has a relative altitude in the hypoxic range (or just below it) before the mission commences.

One conclusion might be that although vital organs are protected from hypoxia to some extent, they are not protected from the effects of hypoxia on the body as a whole. Another way of presenting this would be to state that tissues that are relatively nonvital need to acquire an adequate level of oxygenation for vital tissues to function properly.

A similar approach could be used to explain the symptoms of mountain sickness. The effect of muscular effort in climbing may produce metabolites (when the heart-brain-lung complex has competed for oxygen) that adversely affect cerebration and pulmonary function. Pulmonary edema has been known to occur in previously healthy individuals at as low an altitude as 8000 feet with rapid climbs. A further analogy is the toxic effects of localized injury or infection on the general system without demonstrating a bacteremia or septicemia.

The main point is that a patient does not only need oxygenation of his cerebral and cardiac tissue but for *all* tissue.

Oxygen Delivery Apparatus

A summary follows of the FiO_2 that might be attained by using a variety of respiratory cannulas and masks, with comments on their individual advantages and disadvantages in the aviation environment. The oxygen concentration which each type of mask can provide depends on the flow rates provided through it (Table 18). It also depends on the mask fitting the face and on connecting tubes being fitted correctly without leaks or kinks in the tubing between the flow regulator, humidifier, and the mask.

Table 18.   Oxygen Concentration Abilities of Cannulas and Masks.

Device	$FiO_2(\%)$	Flow Rate (liters/min)
Nasal cannula	25–35	6
	up to 50	8
Simple mask	35	6
	up to 55	10
Laerdal pocket mask	up to 80	15
	up to 50	(mouth to mask at 10 liters/min)
	up to 100	(intermittent occlusion of port at 30 liters/min)
Partial rebreathing mask	up to 60	6–10
Nonrebreathing mask	up to 95	6–10
Dilution masks (Venturi)	24	4
	28	4
	31	6
	35	8
	40	8
	50	12

Oxygen tubes become obstructed more often during the transport of a patient than in a hospital-ward environment.

Nasal Cannulas.   From the patient's point of view, the great advantage of these cannulas is that he can speak, eat, and drink during oxygen administration. They also allow the inhaled gas to be warmed and partially humidified by the nasal lining. The prongs should curve downward for efficient use and to prevent jets of gas from being directed toward the ostia of the frontal sinuses (painful). There is only a slight waste of oxygen during expiration. FiO_2 is capable of providing 25% to 35% at 6 liters per minute.

Simple Mask.   This type of mask has an oxygen inlet and also has exhalation ports on the side of the mask. As the patient exhales, the O_2 flow continues and exits with the expiration gases through the ports. There is some wastage of O_2.

Hudson Mask.   This type is similar to the simple mask, but it has an air dilution inlet at the O_2 inlet. This increases total flow but limits concentration. Some oxygen is wasted on exhalation. Neither the simple mask nor the Hudson mask assist in conserving humidity.

Laerdal Pocket Mask.   The latest version of this useful mask has an oxygen inlet on the side of the mask. It is collapsible and stows easily. Its best use is for mouth-to-mask ventilation in respiratory arrest. The inflated cuff of the present version does not require blowing up before use, which was a nuisance in the earlier models. Larger tidal volumes can be given to a patient using this mask during respiratory arrest than can be given using an Ambu bag and mask. The portal is of a standard size to accommodate demand regulator valves should it be used for positive-pressure breathing. In that instance, the oxygen inlet nipple should be blocked off.
 FiO_2 delivered mouth to mask with an O_2 inflow of 10 liters per minute can provide 50%. With a 30 liters per minute inflow and intermittently occluding the mask port, 100% can be achieved. Used as a simple mask with inflow of 15 liters per minute, 80% can be reached if the patient is breathing spontaneously. In aeromedical care, the mask should not be used routinely for oxygen maintenance if other types are available that do not require such high flow rates. Oxygen disappears rather quickly when flow rates over 10 liters per minute are used.

Partial Rebreathing Masks.   These masks have a bag reservoir and also have exhalation ports. To use properly, the flow must be sufficient to prevent the reservoir bag from completely collapsing on each breath. The first portion of exhaled gas (still O_2-rich as it only traveled in that part of the respiratory tree that did not absorb O_2) reenters the bag to some extent, and the remainder exits through the ports. This not only economizes on the use of oxygen, but also maintains more respiratory water vapor for rebreathing and assists in conserving humidity. An FiO_2 of up to 60% can be achieved with this mask using a flow rate of 6–10 liters per minute.

Nonrebreathing Masks. They are similar to the partial rebreathing masks but have a one-way valve between the mask and the reservoir bag. There are other one-way valves on each of the exhalation ports. This type of mask is the most economical with regard to O_2 consumption when high FiO_2 is required. Expired gas does not reenter the bag, but as the oxygen flow is shut off by a one-way valve during expiration, economy is not reduced to any extent. As all the expired gas exits through the exhalation ports, a considerable amount of humidity is lost. FiO_2 levels are not influenced by atmospheric pressure to any significant extent, which is an advantage when high FiO_2 levels are warranted. However, it is a disadvantage in that the nonrebreathing mask cannot be used if lower FiO_2 levels are indicated. FiO_2 can deliver approximately 95% if the mask fits well and the flow is such that the bag never totally collapses.

Dilution Masks (Venturi). In the U.S., color-coded adapters come with the Venturi masks. Each color indicates the particular oxygen concentration the mask will deliver when used as the adapter. Each adapter is designed for a particular flow rate. Most masks now come with five adapters, some with six (Table 19).

Positive-Pressure Oxygenation. Two distinct circumstances can be considered for the use of positive-pressure breathing. The first is when it is known that a patient will require it during transport. In such a case, the patient must be transported on a respirator and will possibly be using a respirator at the time he is picked up for transport. The second is when the need for positive-pressure oxygenation was not expected, and a respirator is not on board the aircraft. The need for positive-pressure breathing may arise because of some deterioration in the patient's condition or failure of a pressurization system. Intentional loss of altitude may alleviate the need for positive pressure to some extent. An emergency landing might also be considered. However, over the ocean or inhospitable terrain this choice may not be open.

Without a respirator, some positive breathing can be achieved using an Ambu bag, a bag reservoir, and a high flow rate of oxygen. Another method is to use a pocket mask with a good seal to the face; provide a high flow rate of oxygen to the inlet nipple (20 to 30 liters per minute);

Table 19. Venturi Masks.

Adapter Color	Flow Rate (liters per minute)	O_2 Concentration (%)
Blue	4	24
Yellow	4	28
White	6	31
Green	6 or 8 (according to make)	35
Pink	8	40
Orange	12	50

and intermittently occlude the larger port with a finger, removing the finger during exhalation.

Ambu Bags. There are many designs of Ambu bags made of different materials. Each has its own advantages or disadvantages. The Laerdal RFBII is possibly the easiest to use, maintain, and clean. It is transparent and has a capacity of 2000 cc. However, 2000 cc will not be delivered to a patient when the bag is squeezed with the normal hand; approximately half that amount might be delivered under pressure to the respiratory tree. Another reason it cannot be used to replace a respirator for any length of time is that it requires full attention and effort toward respiratory functions and does not leave a hand free to tend to other concerns such as IVs, monitors, vital signs, etc. It is extremely useful for short periods of increased oxygenation when used with a good-fitting mask and a high O_2 flow rate into a reservoir bag.

Respirators. The simplest type of respirator is one using a demand valve regulator, such as the Robertshaw demand valve. The positive-pressure flow can be operated manually by pressing a button on the regulator or can be automatically triggered by a patient's inspiratory negative pressure. Unless positive-pressure breathing is needed in an emergency situation, these demand valve systems should not be used as the means to increase oxygenation over a period of time. The high flow rates waste oxygen, gastric distension soon occurs, and periodic careful maintenance is required for the working parts of the regulator.

A simple respirator which will automatically control respiration for the apneic patient is the PNEUPAC respirator, made by the PNEUPAC Company of Dunstable, England (Fig. 31). It is lightweight, durable to harsh treatment, and effective and easy to operate. It is powered by the gas from the same oxygen cylinder that provides the flow to the patient. It has few moving parts, is adjustable for use by adults and children, and uses only small amounts of oxygen to power it. It can be used with the oxygen cylinders to be found in the U.S. and England, as the code pin

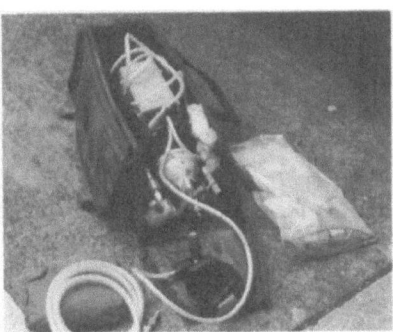

Figure 31.   Pneupac respirator.

fittings are the same. A similar type of unit used in Germany has D.I.N. fittings and is not interchangeable with the U.S. connectors. However, the Pneupac Company makes a decanter adapter which allows a U.S. or English cylinder to be refilled from a German cylinder or from cylinders of other countries that use the D.I.N. type of coding.

The simple respirators which depend on a regulator valve providing positive pressure and do not allow any meaningful control over minute volume, airway pressure, and ventilatory rhythm timing are often termed "resuscitators." For convenience, the more complicated respirators which allow greater control over ventilation might be termed "therapeutic respirators."

Therapeutic Respirators. These machines have gained considerable complexity during the last 10 years. There are numerous models on the market. Each model has its own idiosyncrasies, so that a respiratory therapist must familiarize himself with each new model as the need to operate it arises. It would be courting disaster to send a medical flight attendant on a mission in which the patient's respirator is unfamiliar to him.

It is interesting to report that the degree of complexity is fading with newer models, so that the controls on the panels are more self-explanatory.

Choosing a Respirator (Ventilator). A patient who will require a respirator during his transport must be in such a condition that he will require many other medical accoutrements, all of which have a weight and a volume. If a light aircraft will be used, its useful payload may be between 1500 and 2000 lbs. Two in the cockpit, two attendants, and the patient may well weigh up to 1000 lbs before any equipment or luggage is taken aboard. A flight bag and contents for a critical-care mission will be over 40 lbs; oxygen cylinders might account for 80 lbs; and suction apparatus, IV equipment, and monitor will add another 40 lbs. Stretchers, blankets, mattresses, and other essentials for the patient add on weight, and everyone on board usually has some personal luggage. Therefore, if any respirator is to be used on a mission, it would be wise to choose an aircraft that has a useful payload over 3000 lbs. It really is more a matter of choosing a respirator then choosing an aircraft to accommodate it. Whenever possible, a respiratory therapist should accompany the patient if a respirator is to be used, unless the medical flight attendant is an anesthetist.

Respirators come in many sizes and weights. Some will not even fit into a ground ambulance, and most require electric power. Thankfully, ventilators have become somewhat more compact. A good example of an efficient, compact volume ventilator is the LP 4 made by Life Products Inc. of Boulder, Colorado (Fig. 32). It will operate up to 1 hour on an internal battery or it can operate off a 110 VAC, 60 Hz, 3 amp circuit or a 12 VDC auto-type battery. It has audible alarms which monitor low and high pressures or power failure. The unit weighs 26 lbs, is 8¾" high, 10¾" deep, and 12" wide.

Please note that almost all ventilators have attributes which according to the testing criteria of the School of Aerospace Medicine of the U.S.A.F. make them unacceptable for use in aeromedical transport. Most

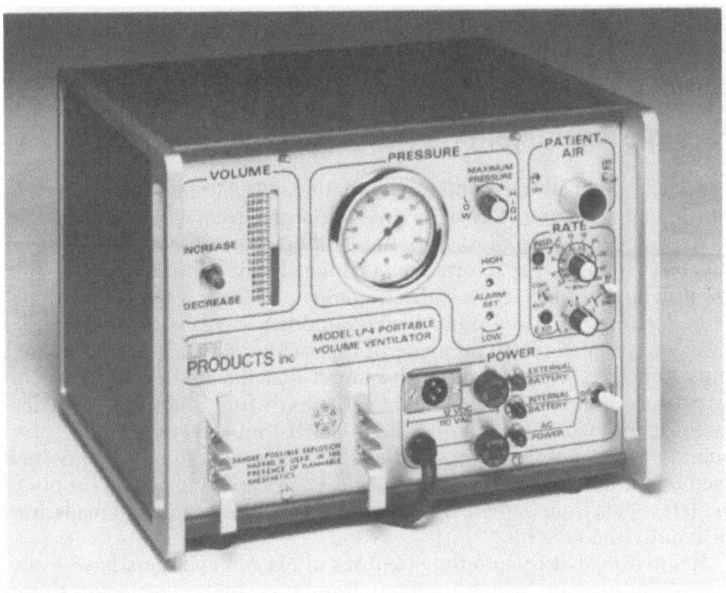

Figure 32. Model LP4 portable volume ventilator. (Life Products Inc., Boulder, Colorado.)

of them give excessive peak airway pressure during rapid decompression. In practice, rapid decompression is not to be expected; should it occur, the patient would be transferred to a simple positive-pressure apparatus until favorable altitude had been reached. Most ventilators also produce excessive EMI, and if a ventilator is to be used repeatedly for aeromedical work it should be modified to reduce the EMI.

Neonatal Respirators. A special category of respirator is used for the transport of infants with such conditions as hyaline membrane disease or prematurity. One unit has been evaluated for in-flight efficiency and shows promise of being valuable in providing high-level care for the critically ill newborn. It is produced by Airborne Lift Support Systems.[4]

Humidification. Humidification is necessary during oxygenation if therapy is to continue for more than a short period. In aircraft with pressurizing systems, the air is rapidly circulated and may be interchanged as frequently as every 2 minutes. This can cause a low cabin humidity. Respirators usually have some humidifying device attached to them. If a humidifying bottle is of the nondisposable type, it must not be used for

[4] From Colton J. S. et al. Air transport of sick infants. Aviat. Space Environ. Med. 50(2):177–181, 1979.

another patient before it has been thoroughly cleaned and fresh water added.

Foreign Equipment

A medical flight attendant on an international flight might be exposed to equipment not seen before or having differences from what the attendant is familiar with. The most important difference is the color-coding of oxygen cylinders. The international code color is white; in the U.S. it is green. The other U.S. color codes for other gases follow the international code. Cylinders must also be checked in other ways than by color code.

When a transfer is to be made of a patient who is already intubated and/or on a respirator, it might be found that the connections of some respiratory tubes do not fit others if they are from different countries. Tubes can be changed before a flight so that all are compatible. Infrequently this is not possible, so an adapter may need to be used. A trick used by the ambulance service of S.A.M.U. in Paris is to carry a supply of the latex teats from baby-feeding bottles. They can be cut and made into an improvised adapter.

Regulators that fit onto the openings of oxygen cylinders have a system of coding pins which prevents lines from being connected to the wrong type of gas. Each gas has its own coding pin arrangement. These differ in parts of the world. A decanter adapter is required to fill a U.S. or English oxygen cylinder from a cylinder having a different coding arrangement.

The Therapist's Performance

Oxygenation of the patient has been addressed, and the effects of hypoxia have been discussed. It must not be forgotten that the medical flight attendant is in the same aviation environment as his patient and is subject to the same degree of hypoxia as the cabin environment presents to the patient. There will be times when the therapist will require therapy. If the attendant is healthy, does not unduly exert himself physically, and the cabin altitude does not exceed 8000 feet, it is unlikely he will require supplementary oxygen. If supplementary oxygen is indicated for the attendant, it must be used to maintain performance.

This might be an opportune place to elaborate further on the medical flight attendant's care of himself. An influence on performance that is almost always present in the aviation environment is *distraction*. This can only be overcome by recognition of the problem and by perpetual guard and mental discipline. The medical flight attendant should feel free to care for himself in all judicious ways to combat any influence that will diminish his ability to care for the patient. It is in the patient's interest. In this respect, forethought to instigate preventive measures is laudable. Clear those nasal passages, empty that bladder, secure the seatbelt, minimize the chance of airsickness and disorientation, use oxygen when indicated, don't smoke or drink before a mission, and enjoy the experience and the privilege of a unique responsibility.

Sudden Decompression

Sudden loss of pressure in the cabin from failure of the pressurization system or from the blowout of a window or a door can cause death from severe hypoxia for all on board if prompt action is not taken. This important subject will be addressed further under Emergencies in the Air.

Scuba Diving and Hyperbaric Chambers

You may wonder why a section on scuba diving should appear in a book on aeromedical care. There are two reasons. The first is to draw attention to the danger of flying within 24 hours of the completion of a dive. For 24 hours, the decompression to sea level or ambient land pressure may not have been completed with regard to reversion of the nitrogen in the tissues to a state in which the formation of embolic bubbles is no longer a danger. After a dive, an individual exposed to altitude (even the 6000 feet of a pressurized cabin as is to be expected on a commercial flight) is in danger of suffering the decompression sickness of diving (the bends) which can lead to serious neurologic deficits and tragedy. The danger is proportional to the altitude experienced and the length of flight time to which exposed. Longer flights (over 30 minutes) increase the danger.

The second reason to mention scuba diving is because the number of persons diving for recreation is increasing every year, and more diving accidents are to be expected. Requests will be received for the air transport of patients suffering from the effects of rapid decompression. The patient is likely to be in places not easily accessible to a hyperbaric chamber (an essential piece of equipment for the successful treatment of the decompression sickness of diving).

Depending on resources available, there are a number of ways of handling a request for aeromedical aid for a patient in trouble because of diving. What should *not* be done is to immediately evacuate the patient by air in an unpressurized aircraft, no matter how low the pilot may think he will be able to fly. If hyperbaric treatment is necessary and not available where the patient is located, a pressurized aircraft can be used if it flies below the altitude at which it can maintain a sea level cabin pressure. The cabin pressure must not be allowed to decrease (or the relative cabin altitude increase).

Small hyperbaric chambers are manufactured that can be carried in some aircraft. The minimum weight of these mobile chambers, with the ancillary equipment and gas cylinders necessary for their operation, is about 600 lbs. The dimensions are such that large doors are needed for the aircraft to allow the loading of the equipment when it is fully assembled.

An alternative method to transporting a patient by air in a hyperbaric chamber might be to fly in the rescue chamber and treat the patient at the site until it is safe for him to be flown without it. Portable chambers have been transported slung below a rotary aircraft. As far as the author is aware, this has not been done while a patient was in the chamber, but it is possible off-shore oil rig operators have used this method. Hyperbaric treatment may be required for a number of days and, if it is at all possible, the patient should be airlifted in a portable chamber to a facility which has a larger unit.

It is also likely that those who have suffered a diving accident will have other injuries as well as those secondary to decompression. These other injuries are more efficiently cared for in a hyperbaric chamber large enough to allow medical personnel to be present with the patient. A company called Environmental Tectonics Corporation (ETC) International (Southampton, Pennsylvania 18966) has manufactured and serviced approximately 200 hyperbaric chambers. The company manufactures two versions of the emergency rescue chamber, one of which is designed to accommodate a medical attendant with the patient. The space for the attendant and the position the attendant must take allows only limited care, but that care is where it is most useful—near the head, the airway, and the upper thorax. Of great importance is the psychological support a close attendant can give a patient under conditions inducive to acute claustrophobia (Fig. 33).

In the U.S. a National Diving Accident Network (DAN) is available 24 hours a day to answer questions on diagnosis, immediate care, transportation, and chamber location for emergency consultation regarding diving accidents.[5]

The service is sponsored by the National Oceanic and Atmospheric Administration, the National Institute for Occupational Safety and Health, and the Department of Energy. The service points out that certain manifestations appearing after diving may require immediate transfer of the victim to a recompression chamber. The manifestations can be

[5] This network can be reached by calling (919) 784-8111 (Duke University Medical Center) or (301) 528-7814 (Maryland Institute for Emergency Services) and asking for DAN.

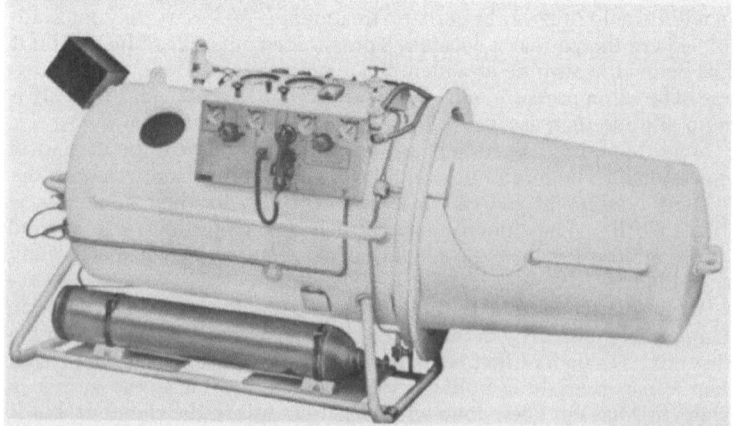

Figure 33.   Bara-Med, Model R-100 hyperbaric chamber. (Courtesy of Environmental Tectonics Corporation, Southampton, Pennsylvania.)

indicative of arterial gas embolism or decompression sickness (bends), as noted below:

Arterial gas embolism: Unconsciousness, paralysis, weakness, confusion, headache, or any other neurological deficit. It can be associated with pneumothorax or air under the skin of the neck. It can result from as shallow as 4 feet of water depth.

Decompression sickness (bends): Joint pain, back or abdominal pain, paralysis, numbness, tingling, inability to control bowels or urine, headache, dizziness, partial blindness, confusion, shortness of breath, chest pain, cough, or shock.

Should any of the above manifestations be elicited in a preflight assessment of a patient requiring air transportation it must be determined whether or not the patient has recently been diving.

Mexico is a popular vacation place for people from the United States and Europe. Many vacationers may try scuba diving there. It is inevitable that some will have accidents and might need hyperbaric treatment.[6]

INTRAVENOUS THERAPY

Need for IV Lines

Intravenous fluids will be required when the oral route of replenishing fluids is not available or is contraindicated. It is rare for a seriously ill or injured patient to be in such perfect fluid balance that he can tolerate 4 or 5 hours without fluids without experiencing some deleterious effect. If vomiting has been one of the symptoms of the medical condition, it is unlikely that symptom will subside or not recur in the aviation environment. Perhaps the surgical nature of the patient's condition may dictate that nothing be given by mouth.

It is desirable, of course, that any hypovolemic state be corrected before a transfer flight. This having been done, the original cause of the hypovolemia should be scrutinized to see if it is more likely to recur in the aviation environment or be aggravated by it. A patient who has had any indication for intravenous therapy during the 24 hours before transfer should certainly be transported with a line running.

Many patients will fall into a category in which their fluid balance is satisfactory and there is little reason to believe it will not stay so on a transfer flight. However, a number of them will be at risk of requiring intravenous medications on an emergency basis. Examples of these situations are patients with convulsive disorders with recent attacks and post-myocardial infarction patients who are symptom-free and in stable condition but are within a few weeks of the infarction and are at risk for

---

[6] There are a number of hyperbaric chambers in Mexico. Those physicians who may require the services of one for a patient might attempt to contact Dr. Hector R. Ramos, an anesthesiologist and expert on hyperbaric treatment, at the Centro Medico Naval in Mexico City (Tel. 550-61-00).

arrhythmias or recurrence if exposed to any hypoxia and excitement. It is judicious to transport this type of patient with an IV line in place or a hep-lock cannula.

Airsickness can be a serious complication for an already-ill patient. Once vomiting has started, oral medications do not have much chance of providing relief. Intravenous medication is the quickest way for an anti-emetic to work. However, the movements of an aircraft cabin at the time of airsickness are not inducive to easy intramuscular injections or intra-venous injections directly into the vein. But even in a "bumpy" cabin, a medical flight attendant can remain secured in a seat and instill medica-tion into an IV line that has medication ports.

The author has only once used an IV line as a means of performing the equivalent of a phlebotomy to relieve pulmonary edema aggravated by polycythemic blood. Applying a venous tourniquet and lowering the almost-empty IV reservoir to the floor, this author removed a beneficial amount of blood from the circulation. This might not be an indication for an IV line, but it does add another use for it should it be in place.

Starting IV Lines

Difficulties can be experienced starting an IV in a light plane in flight, especially during takeoff and climb. It is always difficult when a plane is taxiing, even in large airliners. Whenever possible, an IV should be started before the plane moves and begins taxiing, if one is not already running. If an IV infiltrates or is not running well, an attendant may have to wait until the aircraft is cruising under more calm conditions to rectify the situation.

For a reason to be mentioned later, an IV needle or cannula should not be smaller than an 18-gauge. Choose a site for cannulation that can be secured, and allow some movement of the limb into which it is placed with the least danger of interrupting the flow.

Securing IV Systems

The IV system must be secure:

1. At the IV cannula
2. Along the tubing
3. At the reservoir

Securing the cannula was mentioned above. Attention must be paid to avoid snagging of IV lines on corners, stretcher ends, and other promi-nences, as the light tubing tends to swing around at times. Care must also be taken to see that the tubing is not compressed by the patient, pillow, mattress, or other equipment. The flow-rate chamber must be visible to the attendant and not tucked behind a pillow.

An IV reservoir needs a hook to which the loop on a plastic IV bag or the wire hanging handle of a glass bottle can be attached. If a hook is already present in a convenient location in the cabin, it must be in-spected to see if it is secure enough to hold the reservoir. If the cabin attachment is a ring rather than a hook, a double hook will be required to bridge the cabin ring and the reservoir loop. The possibility of up-and-down jolting or swinging of the reservoir makes it necessary to secure the cabin hook, double hook, and reservoir loop with adhesive tape to prevent dislodgement at an inopportune time. The reservoir can also be prevented from swinging by the use of adhesive tape, but care must be taken not to obscure the fluid level. Glass IV reservoirs should be avoided if at all possible. Special attention must be paid to secure them so that they do not break or hit the patient, the attendant, or anyone else. Protective material cannot be wrapped around the glass bottles, as this would obscure the fluid level.

Factors Affecting Flow Rates

Cannula Size

The size of the needle or cannula can diminish flow, and the smaller sizes are more likely to become clogged if there is any backflow. As there are other reasons why flow may be reduced, it is important to use a needle size 18-gauge or larger on an air transfer.

Constrictions on the Veins Receiving Flow

Possibly the most common cause of reduced flow rate when an IV is running at a preset rate is some constriction occurring above the needle. Bandages that have been used to secure the hand and wrist to a supporting board may constrict the veins, as may clothing around the arm. The flow may be fine with the arm extended, but constriction can occur if the elbow is flexed. This would, of course, be thought of at a hospital bedside. However, in flight, because the aviation environment has some quirks that might reduce IV flow, the more simple reasons for reduced flow may be ignored or temporarily missed.

Constrictions on Tubing

Kinks in the tubing or constriction anywhere along its length can reduce the flow rate. Flow rate is generally controlled by intentionally constricting the tube by some rolling-wheel mechanism, screw clamp, or narrowing-slit plate. IV-giving sets now often come with multiple flow stoppers on the tubing as well as the flow-rate tap. All of these temporary taps must be checked to make sure they do not restrict the flow. Hidden kinks behind pillows and under mattresses must be searched for if a reduced flow rate cannot be explained.

Gravity Head

If an IV reservoir can be hung on the ceiling of an airliner above the level of the overhead storage lockers, the gravity head may be the same as in an emergency department or hospital room. In a light aircraft and even in some of the executive jets, the amount of headroom may limit the gravity head considerably. The reservoir may be only 2 feet or less above the point where the infusion needle or cannula enters the patient. If such is the case, the highest point at which the reservoir can be attached should be chosen.

Pressure Head

The pressure head is related to the gravity head and cannot be raised by elevating the reservoir if it has already been attached to the highest available point. Other methods must be used to increase flow rate by increasing the pressure head, if it is essential the flow rate be increased.

Viscosity of Fluids

When more viscous fluids are being infused, such as blood products, plasma, and some volume expanders, the flow rate may diminish. Everything possible should be done to ameliorate the effects of other causes of reduced flow rate, for when the more viscous fluids are being infused there is usually an important need for them.

Methods of Increasing Flow Rates

Having paid attention to all the factors influencing flow rate and having corrected what can be corrected, any further increase in flow rate must be accomplished by increasing the pressure head of the fluid. The pressure in a plastic reservoir bag can be increased by applying pressure to it circumferentially. In the hospital, this is sometimes done by placing a blood pressure cuff around the bag and pumping it up. There are dangers to this, especially in the aviation environment, as any increase in altitude will cause the cuff to exert increased pressure on the bag because of the expansion of gas with decreased atmospheric pressure. If a pressure cuff is to be placed on the bag, it must have one side made of netting so that the fluid level in the bag can be seen at all times. Air embolus is always a danger when outside pressure is exerted on a reservoir system. The flow of fluid must be frequently checked, and the reservoir fluid level must not be allowed to get too low before the pressure cuff is deflated.

The flow rate of a fluid draining from a plastic IV bag is irregularly influenced by altitude. Bags differ from bottles in that they do not have an air inlet to prevent a negative pressure as the fluid recedes. There is some air above the fluid, but as the fluid recedes, the volume of air remains the same as at sea level and the bag slowly collapses. When the bag is almost full, it is conceivable that the increased volume of the small amount of air would add to the pressure head as it expands with altitude. This, however, is unlikely because of the resilience of the bag wall.

Glass IV bottles compensate for the reduction of fluid volume as the bottle is emptied by having an air-inlet tube (a glass tube from the outside below the inverted bottle) extending vertically up through the fluid to the air space above the fluid. This tube usually has a cotton filter plug at the lower end to filter the air as it ascends into the bottle. Should the plug become wet and act as a seal, it is conceivable the volume of air above the fluid could expand with gain in altitude and increase the flow rate. It rarely does however, and the air above the fluid has a pressure which is balanced with that of the cabin.

The pressure above the fluid can be artificially increased by attaching a pump to the air-inlet tube. This accomplishes the same as applying circumferential pressure to a bag. The same danger of air embolus exists if the fluid level is allowed to drop too low, cannot be seen, and if altitude is gained. There is double jeopardy with glass bottles, as the air expansion occurs above the fluid in the bottle *and* in the restricted cuff if one is used as the source of increased pressure. The safest way to increase flow rate is to manually squeeze a plastic bag reservoir, monitoring the flow rate as it is done and being ever-observant of the fluid level in the bag. In practice, it is safest, more convenient, and less time-consuming to increase intravenous infusion of fluids by intermittently squeezing the bag (in fact, giving a bolus of fluid at specific intervals) rather than attempting to keep a constant higher flow rate. Flow rates can be maintained by placing the bag under a part of the patient (a shoulder, arm, or knee) if the amount of fluid in the bag is checked frequently. For keep vein open (KVO) rates, this is very suitable and overcomes the diminished gravity head that might be hindering the flow.

Prevention of Air Embolus

Wherever IV therapy is being given, there is some danger of air embolus if certain conditions exist. If an IV fluid reservoir becomes depleted and the air in the reservoir has a pressure in excess of the venous pressure at the point of cannulation, air will enter the venous circulation. Precautions to avoid this include changing the bottle or bag before it is depleted of fluid, keeping the point of cannulation below the level of the heart, and (for clear fluids) using a filter to trap any air bubbles. The filters have a membrane 0.2-μm gauge. This precludes their use with blood products and volume expanders with larger molecules and mannitol. When clear fluids such as saline, 5% dextrose, or Hartmann's solution are being used, the filter will extract any air in the line to the patient and vent it to the atmosphere.

IV air-extracting filters will not always be available or practical. The flow rate may have been assisted by some elevation of the cannulation point. In such a circumstance, increased vigilance to the fluid level in the reservoir should be given.

When veins are punctured and cannulated, they are kept at a level below the heart whenever possible to prevent air from entering the hollow of the needle. This is especially important with the larger neck veins and the subclavian vein. If the vein cannot be made dependent, a finger must occlude the needle or cannula opening any time it is not connected to a flow of fluid.

The greatest danger of air embolus is when there is some air under pressure above the fluid level, the reservoir is almost depleted, and the cabin altitude increases. The expansion of the entrapped air can force it into the vein. Whenever increased pressure has been exerted to the infusion force of an IV reservoir, the danger of air embolus is increased.

A medical flight attendant must always be able to see the fluid level in the bag or bottle. It is recommended that increased IV flow be achieved by manual compression of the solution bag rather than with a pressure cuff. This, however, is not possible with a glass bottle.

Care of IV Fluids

Commercially made IV solutions will have an expiration date printed on the container, after which they should probably not be used. Solutions carried in a medical flight bag or stored on aircraft may have been subjected to some extremes in temperature. Solutions differ in the degree to which they are damaged by freezing and overheating. Stored solutions should be frequently checked and the storage conditions overseen to prevent thermal damage, puncture, or breakage of solution containers.

If a flight bag is to be repeatedly used to treat severe trauma cases by infusion of volume expanders, a useful IV fluid to be carried in the bag is Haemaccel. It is an ideal plasma substitute, but what makes it more desirable in aeromedical work is the fact that it is very tolerant of freezing and heating. It is stable for 8 years at room temperature (5 years in the tropics). It gels at 3°C, and freezing does not alter the physiological characteristics of the solution. Warming brings it back to its original state. Another benefit of Haemaccel is that it does not interfere with blood-typing and cross-matching as do some other volume expanders, nor does it interfere with the coagulation mechanism. It also protects the renal system by maintaining diuresis at low arterial renal infusion rates. Cardiac overloading is also not as much of a problem with Haemaccel as with the dextrans because the former is excreted relatively rapidly, with only 5% remaining in the blood after 24 hours.

Haemaccel (or its equivalent under other names) is used extensively in Europe. Unfortunately, it is not yet available in the U.S. The F.D.A. has insisted that it undergo every phase of investigation before it is allowed into the U.S. No company has thus far been willing to meet the enormous expense of carrying out the experimentation (repeating everything that has been done in other countries) necessary for acceptance. Although the author approves of the watchful eye of the F.D.A. protecting us from the dangers of unproved medications, he believes Haemaccel could be approved in the U.S. after clinical testing and after critical study of the animal experimentation that has been performed elsewhere. This would save time and money and not diminish the ability of the F.D.A. to protect the public.

As we face increasing amounts of trauma in the U.S., there is a distinct need for Haemaccel or an equivalent to benefit the public. For those who may use it elsewhere in the world, it comes in a flexible pack of 500 ml that can be squeezed to increase the flow rate. It is unbreakable and collapses as the solution empties.

Monitoring Flow Rates

The many factors that can alter flow rates in the aviation environment have been discussed. These factors are frequently changing in importance in such a way that it is difficult to judge what might happen to the flow rate at any particular moment. For this reason, flow rates must be frequently monitored, and it is advisable to schedule a definite check at least every 5 minutes and continuously just before a reservoir runs out and needs to be changed.

In critical-care units, machines are available to accurately regulate the flow and are usually known as infusion pumps. They are expensive, rely on electrical power, and are unreliable if the IV tubing being used is not exactly the caliber and thickness of the tube for which the infusion pump was designed. They are not recommended for aeromedical care.

Other ways of controlling the flow rate have been designed, most of them in the form of a calibrated tap. One is known as Dial-a-Flow. Tests have shown that these are unreliable in the aviation environment with regard to maintaining the flow at a rate to which the tap is set.

The flow rate is observed as a number of drops per minute. Drip chambers come in many forms. The important piece of information necessary to convert the drops to milliliters is the number of drops per milliliter. A swinging flowmeter can add difficulty to observing the flow and should be prevented from swinging by imaginative improvisation.

CARE OF THE TRAUMA PATIENT

The message requesting air transfer of an injured patient should give some indication of what these injuries are. A distant preflight assessment by telephone or radio before the mission begins will provide further information with regard to the extent of the injuries and other medical factors that warrant consideration. Based on this information, a mission can be organized and the provision of necessary equipment arranged.

One important question should be asked before anything is organized and a mission is flown. The question is: *"Does the patient want to be moved?"* This may seem an unnecessary question, but it is not unusual for many persons to be involved when a request for air evacuation is received: physicians, corporations, relatives, colleagues, and friends. Sometimes all of these persons forget to consult the patient, even though he is able to comprehend and express an opinion. This forgetfulness is rarely intentional but is a result of people's genuine concern for the patient. This seems to happen more with trauma patients than in cases where the patient has purely medical problems.

Bedside Preflight Evaluation

Although a distant preflight assessment has provided certain information about a patient's injuries, a bedside evaluation must be made as though the patient was newly injured. All systems must be examined before the patient is evacuated by air. If a medical flight attendant is unable to leave the aircraft to travel to where the patient is located, the examination will have to be performed in the ambulance as it arrives at the airport.

A medical flight attendant cannot rely fully on any previous diagnoses until confirmatory evidence is obtained. Especially in patients with multiple injuries, it is not difficult to miss the diagnosis of some injuries such as subluxation of the spine and fractures of the pelvis. This does not always reflect on the competence of those who delivered the initial care. Certain diagnoses are easily missed in the acute phase of multiple trauma. Those physicians who do not discover these other injuries days after the initial examination have had little experience with the complexities involved.

The medical flight attendant who is examining a patient some days after an accident has many advantages over the surgeon who gave the initial care. X-rays that are available should be examined and the date they were taken noted. If physical findings do not coincide with the x-ray findings or reports, further x-rays should be ordered if at all possible. If a chest x-ray taken 3 days previously when the patient was admitted does not show a hemothorax but clinical examination on the third day suggests one is present, another x-ray should be taken. If this is not possible, the clinical findings must be relied on.

Relatively simple clinical tests using only the hands of the examiner can demonstrate whether a fracture might be present in the pelvis, if the patient is conscious. This knowledge is very important in patients with multiple injuries. The integrity of the urinary collecting system depends on it to some extent, as does the peripheral circulation to the lower limbs. Of great importance is the danger of exsanguination if fractures of the ilium are missed. A fracture of the ilium, which may not present very remarkable x-ray findings if the angle of projection is not advantageous, can be life-threatening. Ruptured vessels on the anterior surface of the bone may have bled and then temporarily sealed when the blood pressure was low during the first reaction to injury. The seal of these vessels is not very reliable should the blood pressure be raised to a significant extent during transport. Clinical signs negating pelvic fractures allow some reassurance that iliac bleeding will not occur unexpectedly.

If a patient is in coma, pelvic pressure in various axes will not provide much information on whether a fracture is present since the patient is unable to show a response to pain other than pupil-size change. Clear urine from a Foley urinary catheter, adequate femoral pulses of equal intensity and a lack of bruits may be the only clinical signs to take note of unless crepitus is felt. Some have maintained that fractures can be detected by percussion transmitting sounds to other parts of a bone and then heard through a stethoscope. The author has found this of no use for pelvic fractures but has infrequently been able to diagnose a fractured hip by this method. However, the external rotation of the foot gives a better clue.

Good x-rays can be invaluable, but a medical flight attendant on a mission to another country may not find the x-ray services to be the same as found at home. The number of films to be taken for one patient may be strictly limited when one machine and one technician serve a large hospital that may have an outpatient attendance of 800 a day. Therefore, clinical judgment may need to be sharpened in those who have continually had the luxury of unlimited access to radiological and laboratory diagnostic assistance.

Some important questions must be answered before a patient who has suffered multiple trauma is transported by air:

1. Has the patient any injuries that contraindicate air evacuation?
2. Has the patient any conditions or injuries that are unduly affected by altitude?
3. Is the patient's volemic status such that the fluids and equipment carried on the flight can ameliorate significant fluid or electrolyte imbalance?
4. Has the patient sufficient circulating hemoglobin?

5. Is there danger of hemorrhage (of any sort) during the flight?
6. Are any conditions present that might require some active procedure being performed in the air?
7. Will the patient's airway be secure and will means be available to keep the airway patent should vomiting occur?
8. Are there any fractures that have been recently casted?
9. Can fractures be immobilized during transport by some other means than counter weights and air splints?
10. What will be the oxygenation requirements of the patient during transport?
11. Is the intravenous line that is already running in the most appropriate vein for the condition of the patient and the circumstances of the transport? Is the needle or cannula of sufficiently large bore?
12. Is it in the patient's interest to be transported at the time arranged?
13. Reconfirm that the patient wants to be moved.

The Aeromedical Care of Specific Systems

Head Injuries[7]

Whether lucid, comatose, in a postconcussive state, known to have a space-occupying lesion within the skull (either solid or fluid), or recovering from cranial surgery, the *signs and symptoms that mark the level of consciousness and cerebral ability must be noted before the flight.* How this is done and what method is used to record the findings will depend on the training of the attendant. One method of recording both cerebral function and level of consciousness is by using the *Glasgow scale* (Table 20). The scale is based on eye opening and verbal and motor responses as a means of monitoring changes in level of consciousness. It is described here so that those who might be flight attendants can compare it with the method they are presently using and refresh themselves of the elements that should be observed to reach a useful conclusion. The best total of the Glasgow scale is 15. Beyond the signs indicating this full level of consciousness, memory, spectrum of emotions, and cerebral ability to calculate and reason might be noted.

Any changes in the patient's cerebral condition have to be judged on the improvement or deterioration indicated by variations from the pre-flight condition. The medical flight attendant's duties, beyond observing for these changes, are related to:

1. Protecting the patient from stimuli that might increase intracranial pressure
2. Maintaining an adequate airway with sufficient oxygenation to ensure oxygenation of the brain
3. Maintaining a nutritional supply to the brain
4. Preventing injury to paralyzed or insensitive limbs and skin
5. Ensuring a draining outlet for urine
6. Being prepared to deal with convulsions should they occur

With head injuries (if the cardiovascular status and other injuries allow it), the head end of the stretcher should be raised and the head should be forward in the cabin, if cross-cabin placement is not possible.

[7] Including postcranial surgery cases and facial injuries.

Table 20. The Glasgow Scale.

	Value
Eyes	
Open	
spontaneously	4
to verbal command	3
to pain	2
No response	1
Motor Response	
To verbal command—obeys	6
To painful stimulus	
localizes pain	5
flexion-withdrawal	4
abnormal flexion (decorticate rigidity)	3
extension (decerebrate rigidity)	2
no response	1
Verbal Response	
Oriented and converses	5
Disoriented and converses	4
Inappropriate speech	3
Incomprehensible sounds	2
No response	1

Nausea and vomiting are symptoms often associated with cerebral concussion, so a patient with a head injury may be more prone to motion sickness. The strain of vomiting is of no help to cerebral edema already present unless the patient is overhydrated. Anticonvulsants are appropriate before a flight if no contraindications exist. Diazepam is a short-acting anticonvulsant which may alleviate anxiety but may modify cerebration levels.

An injured brain requires more glucose but should be protected from overhydration. An IV of 5% dextrose in water at a slow flow rate is warranted. The IV line may be required for the control of convulsions.

Convulsions Occurring in Flight. The lights, sights, and other stimuli of the aviation environment can be more provocative to a patient having a condition which lowers his convulsion threshold. Such patients may receive anticonvulsant medication before the flight, but a convulsion can still occur. Hypoxia also lowers the convulsion threshold and should be corrected. Should a convulsion occur in flight, it can most often be controlled by giving intravenous diazepam (Valium) in incremental doses of 5 mg repeated every 3 minutes to a total of 15 mg. During a convulsion, the airway should be maintained as well as possible (difficult), and a bite stick should be used to prevent biting of the tongue, lips, or buccal lining. For a varying period of time, the postictal state will confuse the signs and symptoms denoting the level of cerebration.

Caution: Even though a patient gives the impression of being unconscious with regard to sight, hearing, and touch in the postictal state and in some comata, it is well to act as though every word may be heard by the patient. Many physicians and nurses have been embarrassed to later learn that a patient heard and *remembered* what was said in his presence when it was thought he was comatose. Aircraft noises do alleviate this risk to some extent but cannot be relied on.

A recent air encephalogram with air still in the ventricles is a contraindication for air evacuation unless the plane to be used has a pressurized system that will maintain the cabin at a relative altitude equal or almost equal to sea level. The same applies to cases of skull fractures associated with an aerocele.

Facial Injuries

A number of aspects make facial injuries worthy of special care in the air. Facial sinuses may have been damaged and may contain a mixture of blood and air. The trauma or reactive edema may have obstructed the ostia, and the problems associated with gas expansion and contraction in these closed spaces need to be faced.

Distortion of the bones and soft tissues of the face may embarrass the airway. Associated injuries of the larynx (look for subcutaneous emphysema) and the cervical spine (with the orbits and contents) should be looked for. Subcutaneous emphysema will spread with decreased cabin pressure, a missed cervical spine injury may be aggravated during airway modification, and air trapped in the orbit may expand.

Mandibular fractures may have been wired for immobilization with the upper and lower teeth affixed to each other. This presents a hazard should the patient vomit. Some appliance must be handy to release the wires if vomiting cannot be prevented. Such cases should possibly be transported with a nasogastric tube in place so that the stomach can be emptied at frequent intervals. Comatose patients should likewise have gastric drainage.

Eyes

The eye is especially sensitive to hypoxia. The sensitivity is increased by any retinal disease, injury, or increased intraocular pressure. Hypoxia causes increased intraocular pressure. An eye with a perforating injury is at risk of extruding the globar contents if there is a significant drop in cabin pressure. Should the contents not extrude, the damage already present can be aggravated by pressure changes. High oxygenation should be provided to any patient with an eye injury or disease. Consultation with an ophthalmic surgeon should be sought, if at all possible, before transport when the eye is at risk. If any intraocular increased pressure is suspected, care must be taken not to give any drugs that might increase the pressure.

Cervical Spine

Cervical spine fractures and subluxations are best treated by applying traction through skull tongs, with screws into the outer table of the calvarium (e.g., Gardner-Wells tongs). In the hospital, traction is usually produced by weights maintaining tension acting over pulleys. Weights and pulleys cannot be used successfully in aircraft because roll and pitch

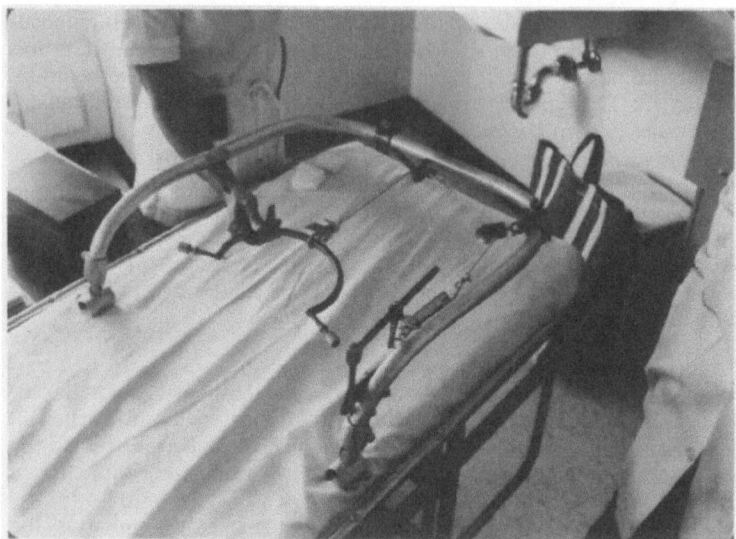

Figure 34. The Rambaud cervical traction frame which attaches to a stretcher and allows the tension of the skull tongs to be controlled and measured on a spring scale.

and forces of acceleration and deceleration tend to swing the weights around, altering the tension of the traction and possibly damaging nearby objects or occupants of the cabin. Chin harnesses can give some traction but have the disadvantage of making airway control more difficult.

Means other than weights must be used to maintain traction. A twisted bundle of orthopedic cord has some resilience when attached directly to the head of the stretcher. Adjustable springs whose tension can be measured by a device similar to a fisherman's scale can be used. An arrangement devised by Dr. Jacques J. Rambaud utilizes a pulley on a frame which carries a cord to a spring scale which, in turn, attaches to a nonsliding ratchet that can be adjusted to the required tension shown on the scale (Fig. 34). The frame is presently only attachable to a regular ambulance stretcher. It could be made to fit a breakaway stretcher or backboard by making the width of the frame adjustable. To counteract movements of the aircraft, rotational stability of the neck must be controlled even when tong traction is applied. This is best done by use of sandbags or tightly rolled towels placed along each side of the head and secured there by wide adhesive tape to the stretcher. On occasions, when turbulence is more severe, the forehead can be taped to either side of the stretcher and will also give more protection from flexion and extension movements of the neck.

A patient with a cervical spine injury having any neurological deficit needs the maximum amount of psychological support that the attendant can provide. Any insensitive areas of the body or paralyzed limbs require close attention to prevent harm. The patient may not know that pressure on some areas may be excessive or that a joint is being strained in a poor position.

Thoracic and Lumbar Spine Injuries
Patients with fractures of these areas of the spine are best transported on a vacuum stretcher if one is available. A backboard, if it is used, will require a 1-inch foam-rubber covering or an egg-crate mattress to alleviate localized, unrelieved pressure. Backboards are uncomfortable enough in normal use on the ground, but the extra pressures that can be experienced in certain attitudes of flight can make them unbearable. Any patient with spinal fractures must be closely observed to see if a paralytic ileus has not caused excessive distension of intestinal loops. Such gaseous distension should be relieved before flight by passage of a nasogastric tube and/or a flatus tube from below. Bladder function should be attended to and, on a long flight, a catheter would be advisable if bladder control is not complete.

Stryker Frame.   Not many light aircraft can accomodate a Stryker frame. Before air transporting a patient on a frame, one must be certain it will enter and fit in the aircraft before leaving the hospital. When multiple moves are contemplated (hospital to ambulance to plane to ambulance to hospital), the complications of each loading and unloading may warrant the patient being removed from the frame and transported on a narrow scoop stretcher with traction attachments. The time taken to make such a transfer from the Stryker to a scoop can save a lot of time at each loading and unloading and allow an aircraft to be used that would not accommodate a Stryker frame. When a Stryker frame is used, arrangements may need to be made to have a lift (elevator) at the airport if the height of the door of the aircraft is higher than manual lifting would reach while keeping the whole frame horizontal.

Thorax
Rib fractures not already associated with hemothorax or pneumothorax and that are not flail or associated with wounds of the chest wall need not cause too much of a problem in flight, but the complications that can occur should be considered. Significant displacement of rib fractures aggravated by excessive thoracic movement or compression from securing devices can cause a pneumothorax to develop. Special care ought to be given to fractures involving the first and second ribs. If fractures are present in these ribs, cervical fractures or subluxations should be carefully looked for, and the neck should be maintained in a neutral position, limiting movement. First-rib fractures are often associated with apical pneumothorax, more extensive pneumothorax, hemothorax, or nerve and vascular injury in the neck. Subcutaneous emphysema may be present which can spread dramatically at altitude.

An unrelieved pneumothorax, even a small resolving one, can increase in extent with increased altitude and hyperventilation. As it increases, recently formed adhesions may be torn and bleeding may occur. A chest tube should be in place and never closed off during flight. A one-way valve, such as the Heimlich valve, should be attached to the chest tube. The finger of a latex glove or a finger cot can be used to improvise a valve. If rubber bands are used to attach these improvised valves to the chest tube, a piece of adhesive tape should secure the rubber band.

If increased respiratory distress becomes apparent, the valve should be checked or should be removed from the tube, and the end of the tube should be placed in a bottle of water. If this indicates that the chest tube is blocked and signs are present that a tension pneumothorax has developed (e.g., distended neck veins, tachycardia, tracheal shift, tympani, and distant breath sounds), the chest should be needled. Should a chest tube appear to be functioning well but respiratory distress is increasing, a pneumothorax on the opposite side should be looked for.

A patient who is intubated on a respirator providing positive pressure may develop a pneumothorax from pleural rupture. This should be looked for and dealt with if hypoxia is apparent, the airway is adequate to both main bronchi, and sufficient oxygen is being supplied under pressure.

Abdomen

If there is any possibility that trauma to the abdomen has been suffered, a nasogastric tube should be in place before a flight. It should not be closed off in the air; when suction is not being applied, a 2 × 2 piece of gauze should be rubber-banded to the open end and a plastic bag attached to cover the gauze, but loosely enough to allow air to escape.

In abdominal trauma, the two main dangers are related to hemorrhage and gas expansion. Hemorrhage can be delayed some days, even weeks, after blunt trauma (from the spleen, mesenteric hematoma, or aortic tear). Consider these dangers during preflight assessment. The volemic status must also be checked and the latest hemoglobin level judged on its relationship to any hemodilution that may have occurred since the test. Any transfusion that is necessary should be completed before transport, if possible. Transfusion flow may be difficult to maintain on loading and at an altitude with a low gravity head.

Hypertension.   Anxiety and a tendency to hypertension in a patient recovering from intra-abdominal hemorrhage may provoke a recurrence of bleeding if the blood pressure is allowed to rise unduly. Small doses of narcotic potentiated by hydroxyzine may be in order to prevent this from happening.

Gas Expansion.   The strain that expanding gas within the intestinal tract can place on suture lines that are not securely healed must be relieved by nasogastric decompression. If preflight evaluation reveals significant amounts of intestinal gas, every attempt should be made to evacuate the gas before transfer by air. In the case of a closed-loop intestinal obstruction, it would be courting the danger of perforation should the patient be subjected to reduced atmospheric pressure. If there is any suspicion of an intestinal obstruction, a flat and erect x-ray of the abdomen should be taken as part of the preflight assessment, if x-ray facilities are available.

Colostomy.   With a colostomy, an increase in bowel elimination can occur because of the peristaltic stimulation of expanding bowel gas. If air has already been passed into the colostomy bag in flight and there is an increased amount of fecal material in it, changing the bag without leakage may be difficult. It is possibly better to release some of the gas first by making a small vent hole with a needle and covering the hole with a dry Band-Aid. The patient should have a clean, empty colostomy bag before transport.

Pelvis
Undisplaced or minimally displaced fractures of the pelvis usually present no serious problems if they are recognized, pain is relieved, and the patient is handled with care. Vacuum stretchers are the most comfortable and offer the most protection. When more severe fractures are present, consideration must be given to internal injuries to the genitourinary tract, bowel, and iliac vessels and their branches. A retaining urinary catheter should be draining and not closed off. This is for the patient's comfort and to be able to observe the amount and nature of the urine.

Extremities
Before any patient with fractures or soft-tissue injuries of the extremities is transported, the integrity of the blood vessels and peripheral nerves must be inspected. If limbs have been newly casted, it is advisable that the casts be bivalved if the transfer will take more than 30 minutes in the air. This is especially important if a fracture was compound and there may be air in the wound or trapped under the plaster.

After the fracture patient has been secured to the aircraft stretcher, every effort should be made to elevate any limb having distal fractures. Air splints should not be used in flight unless they are constantly adjusted to prevent excessive circumferential pressure. If any fractures are receiving traction through pulleys and weights, an alternative method of immobilization has to be supplied. Loading and unloading and turbulent movements aloft can be expected to transmit some pain-provoking movement to fractures under traction. Gentleness can help, but analgesics would be welcomed by the patient and beneficial for his condition.

Ear, Nose, and Throat
Barometric effects on the ears and sinuses have been addressed earlier. The vestibular apparatus and motion sickness will be discussed later under airsickness.

Epistaxis. Whether from trauma or other causes, a recurrence of epistaxis in flight can be troublesome. A patient transported with nasal packs has guaranteed blockage of nasal ostia. If at all possible, the nasal packs should be removed before flight and bleeding points controlled by cautery. This does increase the risk of recurrence of epistaxis, and simplified means of controlling it must be anticipated. Should bilateral nostril compression for more than 4 minutes not control the bleeding, the nose may need to be repacked. This is rarely easy in flight if lengths of vaseline gauze or hemostatic material are to be used.

Another method is simple, easy to perform, and can maintain a nasal airway. This is by using Merocel nasal tampons (Fig. 35). The tampons come in a compressed, dehydrated state; in this state they are easy to insert into the nostrils. The body fluids from the nasal lining or the blood expand the tampon to fill the nasal cavity. One type has a tube embedded

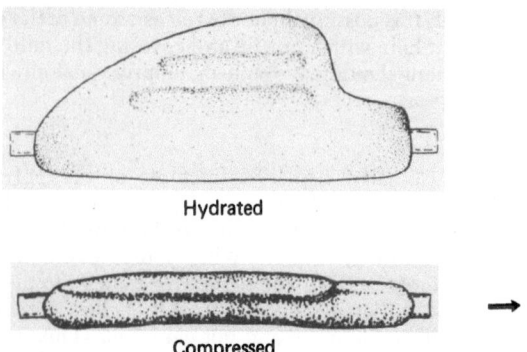

Hydrated

Compressed

Figure 35.   Merocel nasal tampon.

through its length so that air can travel through it to the nasal pharynx. The material is a biocompatible open-cell sponge which has no cellulose of loose fibers that could adhere to the wound in a blood vessel. The tampons are made by the Americal Corporation, Mystic, Connecticut and are marketed under the trade name Merocel.

Tympanic Membrane.   If traumatic myringitis is present and a perforation is apparent, air may have free access should pressure changes in the middle ear cause air movement. It is advisable to filter any air that may enter the perforation. This can be accomplished by taping a loose cotton ball over the external ear. A cotton wick inside the external auditory meatus (should it become moist) would be a barrier for air movement and would hinder a flow of blood should bleeding occur.

Burns
Severe burns will be a frequent cause for the air transport to a distant, specialized burn unit.

Nonemergency Transport of the Burn Patient.   If a patient is hospitalized somewhere in the world where there are adequate facilities to treat serious burns, it is appropriate that he remain there until conditions are stabilized and definitive treatment has been completed. At that stage in treatment, the patient (or those responsible) may request that he be transferred to a hospital nearer to home that is able to care for him during his long convalescence. Such a transfer can be planned without haste, and enough time can be taken to competently meet the requirements of the mission. Needs can be listed with regard to fluid requirements, respiratory support, medications for the relief of pain and anxiety and the control of infection, and means of collecting and measuring urinary output. These missions can be well-coordinated with those who have cared for the patient, those who will attend him during transfer, and those who will receive him into their care.

Emergency Transport of the Seriously Burned Patient.   Transfer of a severely burned patient from an inadequate facility which cannot provide the standard of care necessary to postpone a preventable morbid outcome is a completely different matter from the transfer of a convalescing burn patient. This situation requires fast organization of personnel, equipment, and transport means, and a predesigned plan adaptable to varying degrees of seriousness.

Personnel and Aircraft. To accomplish an emergency transfer of a seriously burned patient, a team of medical flight attendants should be chosen to include:

1. A surgeon who is an expert in burn care
2. An emergency physician experienced in aeromedical care
3. A critical-care nurse from a burn unit

The surgeon and nurse should preferably be from the unit to which the patient is to be transferred.

For transfers of less than 250 miles, a helicopter should be used. If the receiving hospital or dispatching hospital has a heliport or grounds suitable for conversion to a landing pad, transport time and trauma is much reduced. If not, a ground ambulance vehicle will also be needed at one or both ends of the mission. Ground ambulances or helicopters (if practical) will be needed to and from airports if a transfer is to be over 250 miles and will utilize fixed-wing aircraft.

If ground is to be used near the hospitals as improvised helipads, an operations officer and the pilot will advise the hospital authorities of the necessary preparations of the area and the precautions to be followed.

When a helicopter is the only aircraft to be used, it may not be possible for the team of three to accompany and attend the patient on the transfer flight. However, the full team should be sent out with the helicopter to the dispatching hospital to provide the necessary evaluations and preparations for flight. If a tracheostomy needs to be performed by the surgeon, and the patient is put on a respirator, a respiratory therapist should be on the team accompanying the patient.

When a team member has been left behind at the dispatching hospital because of lack of cabin space, that member should be responsible for the communication of all information that will be useful to the receiving hospital. He should also be responsible for the return of any equipment that did not accompany the flight. He may be required to escort the family of the patient to the receiving hospital by other means of transport.

Equipment, Supplies, and Drugs. What will be required to be flown to the patient with the burn-care team will be determined from the answers to the following questions:

1. What is the patient's sex, age, weight, and height?
2. What type of burn was suffered (chemical, thermal, or electrical)?
3. Extent of burns related to surface area?
4. Depth of burns?
5. Which areas of the body are burned?
6. Are there any circumferential burns?
7. Is there any respiratory involvement?
8. Are there any other injuries?

Table 21. Checklist of Equipment, Supplies, and Medications for Burn Victims.

1. Respiratory support
   Airways
   Cannulas
   Masks
   Oxygen
   Positive-pressure appliances
   Respirator
   Humidifier
   Suction
   Tracheostomy set
   Laryngoscopes ⎱ adaptable power
   Bronchoscopes ⎰   source

2. Fluid replacement
   IV-giving sets
   IV needles, cannulas, and
      catheters
   CVP catheters and measuring
      device
   Cutdown surgical sets
   IV fluids
      Crystalloids
      Solutions
      Electrolytes
      Volume expanders, artificial
      Plasma
      Blood
   Means to pressurize IV
      reservoirs

3. Wound Care
   Dressings
   Burn sheets
   Medicaments
   Surgical instruments
   Gowns, gloves, masks

4. Eye Care
   Dressings
   Medicaments

5. Urinary Output
   Catheterizations sets
   Retaining catheters
   Measuring and collecting
      devices
   Medicaments
   Urine testing tape and
      hygrometer

6. Cardiovascular Support
   Montior
   Drugs

7. Peripheral Vascular Integrity
   Surgical Instruments

8. Gastro-Intestinal Support
   Gastric and Nasogastric tubes
   Oral toilet equipment and
      medicaments
   Tube-feeding solutions

9. Prophylaxis/Treatment of
      Infection
   Immunizational injectibles
   Anti-infective drugs, IV, IM
   Gowns, gloves, masks

10. Comfort
    Drugs for pain relief
    Sedatives
    Antiemetics
    Stretcher

11. Maintenance of Body
       Temperature
    Sheets
    Blankets
    Foil blankets

9. What preburn medical conditions existed?
10. What is the known past medical history, including any history of allergies or sensitivity to medication?
11. What is the patient's level of consciousness?
12. What urinary output is being maintained?
13. What sort and amount of fluids have already been given?
14. What medications or biologicals has the patient received?

15. What are the results of any pathological or radiological investigations?
16. What is the patient's religion?

From the answers, the surgeon should be able to advise those at the dispatching hospital on what preparations they should make for the reception of the team and the transfer, keeping the advice within the capabilities of those advised. He should also be able to determine what equipment, supplies, fluids, and medications should be flown out with the team (Table 21).

AIRBORNE CARDIAC CARE

Coronary Artery Disease and Air Travel

Before discussing the care of cardiac patients during aeromedical transfer, some comments on the effect of the aviation environment on those with coronary artery disease might be in order.

The recommended maximum relative altitude for the pressurized cabins of airliners was reduced from 8000 to 6000 feet above sea level only a few years ago. This was done on the basis of repeated reports that the higher of the two altitudes was not being tolerated by older passengers with arteriosclerotic heart disease. As far as the author is aware, no statistics were made public at the time of the change to indicate the extent of the intolerance in terms of attacks of congestive heart failure or outright infarctions. One can only assume the statistics gave enough evidence that altitudes over 6000 feet had been shown to be harmful to some passengers.

One may wonder how much hypoxia is required to precipitate the symptoms of coronary ischemia which in turn might provoke panic and the circumstances for infarction to occur. Some of the circumstances are:

1. The presence of silent or overt anxiety from the flying experience
2. Eating relatively large meals when the digestive system has not already completed its work on a previous meal, diverting blood to the splanchnic system
3. Aerated drinks aggravating gastric distension with elevation of the diaphragm and reduced available pulmonary volume
4. A seating arrangement that does not encourage movement of the legs, causing hypostatic edema and stasis (acidotic blood waiting to be returned to the circulation)

A cabin altitude of 8000 feet may present a level of hypoxia beyond the passenger's tolerance; 6000 feet might be too high for some. Sea level is too high for some who never fly! (350,000 victims die of heart attacks outside of hospitals each year in the United States).

As we are presently having to make some judgments from meager anecdotal information, the author might be excused for mentioning his own experience.

The author is an emergency physician. It is his habit when treating a heart attack victim to seek the patient's flying history. On at least four occasions during the last 7 years, a history was elicited that the patient had flown within the previous 2 days. Two had noticed symptoms in flight that could have been the prodromal symptoms or an actual infarct occurring. (It should not have to be stressed that valid opinion cannot be derived from anecdotal information. However, in the absence of established data on the incidence of heart attacks in the air, hints as to what that incidence might be should not be ignored.)

In light of the above discussion, it should not be surprising that controversy continues as to when, after an acute myocardial infarction, a patient can be safely transported by air. Opinions range from 5 to 26 weeks. Many factors have to be considered: the nature of the heart attack, extent of infarct, position of infarct in the ventricle, preinfarct condition, postinfarctive course, age, sex, medications to maintain compensation and rhythm, cardiac reserve, stability of coagulation system, biochemical levels in the blood, and mental stability. The list is not complete.

A physician will have to make the decision as to whether to transfer the patient by air. The motives behind the request for transfer must be examined. The cardiac care available at the location from which the patient wants to be moved will also color the decision considerably. Each request must be judged on the individual circumstances.

Recommendations[8]

A patient who has suffered a heart attack should not be aeromedically transferred within 1 week of the onset of the acute attack, or less than 1 week after significant arrhythmia has been controlled, or congestive heart failure has resolved, or if still suffering episodes of cardiac pain—except in exceptional circumstances when it is clearly in the patient's interest to be moved by air. Whenever a patient who is suffering from or convalescing from an acute heart attack is transferred by air within 8 weeks of the episode, the transfer should be made:

1. In a pressurized aircraft.
2. The relative altitude of the cabin should never exceed 6000 feet.
3. Advanced cardiac life-support equipment and drugs should be on board.
4. The patient should be connected for cardiac monitoring.
5. An intravenous infusion line should be running or a heplock needle should be in place in a vein.
6. Supplementary oxygen should be provided at all altitudes.
7. The patient should be attended by medical personnel skilled in advanced cardiac life support (preferably two attendants).
8. Preflight sedation should be administered if not contraindicated.

It may be impractical for all cardiac patients to be escorted by a physician trained and experienced in advanced cardiac care as defined by the

[8] These recommendations are those of the author, do not represent any established concensus of opinion, and should not be regarded as representing a minimal standard of care to be imposed on the responsibilities of individual physicians. They are intended to encourage debate that might mollify what controversy now exists, and they were formulated with that intention in mind.

American Heart Association. Flight nurses and technicians may have to provide advanced care including drug therapy, the use of adjuncts for airway control and ventilation, recognition and correction of arrhythmia, and the use of a defibrillator. In such cases, advanced cardiac life support (A.C.L.S.) should be given in accordance with the protocols established by the medical director of the mission. There may be times when medical direction can be given by two-way voice contact through radio transmissions and, in some cases, with telemetry.

The Chance of Need for Resuscitative Procedures in Flight

The need to apply A.C.L.S. on a resuscitative basis in the air is a remote possibility when a cardiac patient is being transferred from one sophisticated medical center to another on a well-planned mission. However, it becomes a real possibility if a patient has suffered a heart attack in some remote place in the world or where adequate cardiac care is unavailable, and he is to be evacuated by air. It may be in the patient's best interest, within the choices open to him, to be evacuated in the acute or subacute phase. Even in these cases, the need for resuscitative measures in flight can be greatly reduced by sensible preflight care.

Cardiac Preflight Preparation

Care in the air will most often be based on a continuation of the cardiac care already given. What that premission care has been should be well known, as should the full history of responses (and lack of responses) to various therapies. Preflight cardiac evaluation, the correction of conditions likely to be detrimental to the patient's cardiovascular status, and the cardiac care to be given during flight all depend on the same tenets.

Tenets of Cardiac Care

Cardiac care is directed toward the prevention and correction of hypoxia, unnecessary hypercapnia, and metabolic acidosis; to maintaining perfusion through sufficiently forceful myocardial contractions at an effective and regular rate; the compensation of congestive heart failure; and the relief of pain and anxiety.

Protocols

The protocols that follow are those of the author and are intended to serve only as a reference for medical directors developing or modifying their own protocols and standing orders.

Preflight Cardiac Evaluation

Whenever practical, preflight evaluation should ideally accumulate data reflecting the patient's condition within the few hours before transport. A night-before assessment may not be valid on the morning of the flight. The data should come from:

1. Physical examination
2. EKG and rhythm strip
3. Fluid balance measurements
4. Blood count

5. Electrolyte balance report
6. Blood gases
7. Chest x-ray

No laboratory, x-ray, or EKG should substitute for a hands-on physical examination. The location of peripheral edema; the quality of heart and breath sounds; and any pain, discomfort, or mental problem will not be seen on the x-ray or discerned in the blood.

Preflight Sedation
Medication may be chosen and ordered by the patient's attending physician. He should be influenced to choose a drug which has antiemetic properties, such as hydroxyzine hydrochloride (Vistaril) 25 mg IM → q 2 h prn up to 3 doses on flight under 6 hours; prochlorperazine (Compazine) 5 mg IM → q 3 h prn up to 2 doses on flight; or diphenhydramine (Benadryl) 50 mg IM → q 4 h prn up to 2 doses on flight.

Preflight IV Setup
Secure heplock needle in vein or IV 5% dextrose in water KVO

Preflight Monitor Connection
1. Place adhesive chest electrodes compatible with leads of monitor to be flown.
2. Check monitor and write-out.
3. Check batteries, including spares.

Preflight Oxygenation Check
Know estimated transport time and estimate oxygen volume requirements, allowing reserve for possible refueling stop. Provide reserve cylinder dedicated for the provision of 100% FiO_2 in resuscitation situation. Connect it (uncracked) through a flow regulator to a Laerdal pocket mask inlet nipple.

Inflight Care
Before using any drugs, the possibility of incompatibility should be considered, such as:

1. Precipitation reaction of furosemide (Lasix) with meperidine (Demerol, Pethidine).
2. Precipitation reaction of morphine sulfate with calcium chloride.
3. Inactivation of epinephrine (Adrenaline) by sodium bicarbonate.
4. Verapamil should not be used if the patient has received propranolol, though recent information suggests there are less dangers than first thought.

A drug given intravenously should be flushed into the circulation by temporarily increasing the flow rate. An interval of time should then be allowed to pass before an incompatible drug is intravenously injected (if it must be given).

Before using a defibrillator, the cockpit crew must be informed so that radios and other electrically sensitive instruments can be turned off during the shock.

Care in Flight

Set up a portable altimeter so that cabin relative altitude can always be seen. Before takeoff, set the altimeter to show readings above sea level. The pilot will inform you of the height of the airport above sea level.

Observations[9]

1. *Blood Pressure:* If systolic and diastolic sound changes cannot be heard, palpate the radial pulse for systolic pressure and observe change in swing of aneroid needle for approximate diastolic pressure. Make a mental note of the force of the pulse to light pressure.

2. *Pulse rate and rhythm*

3. *Heart rate and rhythm:* It should never be assumed that the ventricular rate, as seen electrically on the monitor, is the same as the ventricular rate palpated at the apex or heard there with a stethoscope. Nor should the radial pulse be assumed to be the same as the apical rate. The peripheral pulse (radial or femoral) should be palpated first, then compared to the apical pulse. In arteriosclerotic patients it is sometimes possible to *see* arterial pulsations at the temple or in the brachial fossa. If there is a pulse deficit or arrhythmia is apparent, the cardiac monitor should be turned on. (On longer flights, battery supply may not allow continuous EKG monitoring.)

4. *Ventilatory efficiency:* This can be judged by the ease, rate, and depth of respiration; the color of the skin and mucus membranes; and cerebral changes. If any signs point to a deficiency, corrective action should be taken and the wave form of the monitored EKG noted to see if change has occurred to indicate myocardial ischemia (diminished or inverted T waves, if previously upright).

5. *Chest pain:* This is the most important sign of ischemia or problems ahead. Analgesia should be provided and oxygenation increased. Moderate angina pain should be treated with sublingual nitroglycerin tablets (0.4 mg every 5 minutes to 3 doses). More severe pain, especially if associated with anxiety, should be treated with IV narcotics, such as meperidine 25 mg IV q 10 min prn up to 4 doses. Morphine sulfate may be used in titrated doses of 5 or 10 mg IV, but should probably not be used if any significant bradycardia is present. In the author's experience, the emetic index of meperidine is less than that of morphine, judging from laundry bills.

6. *Congestive heart failure:* Attempt to note the onset (tachycardia, distended veins, and increased respiratory rate) before the onset of frank pulmonary edema. *Caution:* Although congestive heart failure is usually associated with tachycardia, it can occur with a normal pulse rate or a bradycardia in those patients medicated with propranolol. If meperidine or morphine has not already been given, one or the other might be given, followed at an interval by furosemide 50 mg IV. The patient should be propped up in the sitting position (if he is not already). On an ambulance stretcher, it is impossible to lower the legs advantageously. In lieu of lowering the legs, loose venous tourniquets can be applied to the thighs if other therapies have not sufficiently relieved the pulmonary edema.

---

[9] Noise and movement can hinder these observations.

The patient may require digitalization, but it should be withheld if possible if there is any probability of deterioration of the condition that might lead to cardiac arrest. Digitalization should only be done on a medical director's order.

7. *The EKG monitor:* On all but flights of under 1 hour, batteries may need to be conserved and continuous monitoring may not be feasible although desirable. Therefore, monitoring and write-out records should be reserved with specific indications: (a) before taxiing (for baseline and monitor check); (b) after climb-out (to check effects of takeoff and climb); (c) 10 minutes after level-off (to check effects of cabin altitude); (d) during descent before final approach (to check whether any changes need correction before the deceleration of landing); and (e) when any significant change in rhythm occurs, as discerned clinically.

Handling of Unwelcomed Changes in Rhythm

Sinus Tachycardia. (Pulse rate of over 110 per minute, sustained for more than 5 minutes.)

1. If provoked by anxiety—sedation (hydroxyzine or diazepam)
2. If provoked by pain—narcotic (dose-adjusted by considering potentiating actions of recently administered drugs)
3. If due to congestive heart failure—treat congestive heart failure

Supraventricular Tachycardia. (Pulse rate of 160 to 240 per minute.)

1. Treat as soon as possible (on the ground, the rhythm may be tolerated for some time by a previously healthy individual; with aviation factors and known heart disease, decompensation can occur quickly).
2. Attempt carotid massage while watching monitor.
3. Verapamil 5 to 10 mg IV if patient has not recently been on propranolol (fortunately, supraventricular tachycardia is less likely to occur on propranolol).
4. If recently on propranolol, diazepam 5 mg IV, followed by edrophonium HCl (Tensilon) 8 mg IV.
5. If still no conversion and condition deteriorating, prepare lidocaine drip (2 g in 500 cc 5% dextrose in water) and have a bolus ready (75 mg lidocaine); attempt cardioversion (electrical) at less then 50 joules (synchronized).
6. In the event ventricular fibrillation follows, turn off synch and immediately defibrillate at 200 joules (making sure patient is not conscious and rhythm shown is not artifactual).

Bradycardia. With a pulse rate above 40 per minute and no change in stability, check oxygenation and have patient move arms and legs. If no response, pulse below 50 per minute, and signs of decreasing stability, give atropine 0.5 mg IV repeated in 5 minutes prn. Note that any deleterious changes in rhythm may be secondary to hypoxia. When rhythm changes occur, check cabin altitude and oxygenation being provided. If cabin altitude is excessive, request pilot to lose altitude until cabin pressure is acceptable, if maneuver is practical (it might not be over a mountain or above severe turbulence).

First-degree Heart Block. Miss dose of digoxin or quinidine, if due, and check oxygenation.

Second-degree Heart Block. Mobitz I, Wenckebach—treat if ventricular rate is below 50 per minute and patient is hypotensive. Give atropine 0.5 mg IV × 2 q 5 min prn.

Mobitz II AV Block. Double-check oxygenation and cabin altitude. (This dangerous rhythm must be treated, but the treatment may provoke a tachycardia with increased tissue-oxygen requirements in a heart already with some damage.) Give atropine 0.5 mg IV × 2 q 5 min prn and isoproterenol (Isuprel) infusion (1 mg in 250 cc 5% dextrose in water) as ordered by the medical director.

Third-degree Heart Block (Complete Heart Block). Same as for Mobitz II, attempting to maintain ventricular rate around 60 per minute.

Atrial Flutter

Check oxygenation and cabin altitude. If there is a fast ventricular rate which cannot be tolerated by the patient for any length of time, it should be treated. Give digoxin 0.5 mg IV or DC countershock at low joules (20 to 30) after IV diazepam 5 mg.

Choices of therapy might depend on how much time remains of the flight. If 3 hours more flying time is expected and the patient is already in trouble with a persisting atrial flutter with a fast ventricular rate, electrical cardioversion might be more appropriate before digitalization. The procedure is more likely to succeed, and digitalization may add problems later in the flight.

Atrial Fibrillation

Check oxygenation and cabin altitude. Treat the same as atrial flutter, if fast ventricular rate persists and patient is not tolerating the rate.

Ectopic Beats

All ectopic rhythms need not be treated; those that are infrequent and those that are habitual may not require any care other than observation. Some patients have chronic premature ventricular contractions, sometimes with a frequent character, and are symptomless. The previous history is important and can be somewhat reassuring.

The author once transported a young engineer from South America to London who had head injuries and who displayed multiple PVCs on the monitor during the preflight assessment which continued without modifications. During the 2-day preflight observation period, the character of the PVCs never altered, and there appeared to be no effect on his cardiovascular stability. The PVCs were not treated, and information received later showed that he had had the arrhythmia since childhood, though he was not aware of it himself. This transfer is well-remembered because of other worries that arose: an attempted ambush on the way from the hospital to the airport, and the loss of power from one engine causing an unplanned landing on a small island in the Caribbean.

Premature Atrial Contractions. Check oxygenation and cabin altitude. Discontinue or avoid sympathomimetic drugs and stimulants. Frequent PACs with a fast ventricular rate may respond to small doses of propranolol (0.1 mg test-dose first, then 1 mg IV over 5 minutes). There is, however, considerable risk of giving the propranolol if the patient has recently had an acute myocardial infarction. Experience has not been wide with the use of Verapamil in PACs of a frequent nature at a fast total ventricular rate, but it seems promising and may prove to be the drug of choice if the PACs demand treatment in an emergency situation. The dose would probably be between 5 and 10 mg IV.

Premature Ventricular Contractions. It is the change in frequency, or the change in nature (from unifocal to multifocal) of the PVCs that dictates whether they require treatment. Where there have been no PVCs, and they then occur at a rate of more than 8 per minute or a bigemini rhythm appears: check oxygenation and cabin altitude, and give an IV bolus of lidocaine 75 mg with a further 25 mg after 5 minutes, followed by an infusion of lidocaine at 1 to 4 mg per minute.

Unwelcomed and Morbid Rhythms (Ventricular Tachycardia, Ventricular Fibrillation, and Asystole)

A patient with ventricular tachycardia will die within a short time if the rhythm is not corrected. A patient with ventricular fibrillation or asystole is very soon clinically dead unless basic life support is given and the rhythm is converted to one compatible with life.

Ventricular Tachycardia. For short runs where there is no loss of consciousness, treat same as for frequent PVCs. If no response, give bretylium 500 mg in 50 ml injected slowly IV. If the condition is sustained with loss of consciousness, inform cockpit crew that the defibrillator will be used, then ascertain when radios and radio-navigational equipment have been turned off. *Meanwhile try precordial thump.* Now treat in the following sequence:

1. Countershock with synchronization 100 joules × 2 prn.
2. Countershock without synchronization if ventricular fibrillation supervenes.
3. IV lidocaine bolus 75 mg.
4. CPR for 3 cycles.
5. Countershock 100 joules; second shock 200 joules.
6. Bretylium 250 mg undiluted given rapidly IV.
7. CPR for 3 cycles.
8. Same as for ventricular fibrillation.

Ventricular Fibrillation. If this condition is apparent on the monitor and the patient is conscious, check monitor leads. If the patient is arrested with no pulse or heart sounds (if patient is being attended in the air, it must be assumed the arrest was witnessed), proceed as follows:

1. Inform pilot the defibrillator is to be used; try precordial thump.
2. Countershock × 3 prn (100 joules, 200 joules, 300 joules).
3. CPR for 3 cycles.

4. Epinephrine 0.5 mg IV.
5. CPR 1 cycle.
6. Sodium bicarbonate 50 mEq IV.
7. CPR 3 cycles.
8. Countershock × 3 prn (200 joules, 300 joules, 400 joules).
9. Lidocaine 100 mg bolus.
10. CPR.
11. Countershock 400 joules.
12. Bretylium 500 mg undiluted rapidly IV.
13. Countershock.

Note: In no way should the preceding information be used in a cookbook fashion; it should only used as a guide to give some idea of the order of various modalities. How and when they are used will depend on their availability at a particular moment. Defibrillator batteries do have a limit to the number of countershocks they can provide. When thought is given to the rapidity needed for some modalities to have any chance of success, the disadvantage of having only one medical attendant for the patient is glaring.

Asystole.   For any chance of success in the treatment of cardiac arrest with asystole, all intravenous medications that are given must be preceded and followed by CPR to circulate those medications. Asystole includes electrical and ventricular standstill *and* ventricular standstill with electrical activity (electromechanical dissociation). Treat in the following sequence:

1. Precordial thump.
2. Notify pilot that defibrillator might be used.
3. CPR.
4. IV epinephrine 1 mg push.
5. CPR.
6. IV atropine 1 mg push.
7. CPR.
8. IV dexamethasone 20 mg.
9. CPR.
10. Countershock 300 joules.
11. Alternate 2 more doses of epinephrine and atropine.

Cardiopulmonary Resuscitation on Board
Light Aircraft

If cardiac intensive care may be needed in flight, an aircraft should be chosen that has enough cabin space to allow the attendant to perform CPR in the usual manner. However, circumstances may necessitate giving CPR in the confined space of a small, light aircraft. The space in the cabin is such that the roof curves over the patient on the stretcher, leaving little or no room above the patient for reasonable chest compressions. The patient has to be dragged onto the cabin floor where he may be in the groove between the seats. If there is not enough space between the seats for a kneeling attendant, compressions must be applied by leaning over the head of the patient. When two-man CPR is being performed, the rescuer giving the chest compressions might consider giving the compressions with the heel of the foot (unbooted) while bracing the hands against the cabin walls or roof. Under any circumstances, CPR is difficult in an aircraft. Everything possible should be done to prevent its need: good preflight assessment, preparation, and care; the prompt correction of unwelcomed arrhythmias; and the continuous maintenance of adequate oxygenation in an environment not allowed to reach levels of decreased pressure harmful to the patient in his particular circumstance.

Artificial Pacemakers

Complications that Can Occur with Pacemakers

1. *Failure of sensing:* In demand pacemakers, this is commonly due to a low QRS amplitude. It can also be due to a failing battery or the sensitivity control being set too high. A permanent pacemaker battery cannot be changed in the air. The sensitivity control can be turned down on a temporary pacemaker. Inotropic agents (e.g., β_1 effect of isoproterenol) may increase the amplitude of the QRS complex.

2. *Oversensing* can be due to extraneous signals that may be from a loose connection in the pacemaker or the intermittent separation of a broken wire. They can also be from electromagnetic fields, stray electric currents, and undue manipulation of the connecting cable. All these reasons have more chance of occurring in the aviation environment of electric circuits and radio transmissions.

3. *Failure to pace* may be due to poor position of the catheter electrode or to battery depletion causing insufficient current to stimulate a contraction of the ventricle. Isoproterenol may increase the sensitivity of the myocardium so that a smaller current will cause capture.

4. *Dysrhythmias from pacemakers:* Electrode catheters can induce irritation of the myocardial wall causing ventricular arrhythmias. Any of these arrhythmias are more likely to occur if hypoxia, metabolic acidosis, or excessive sympathetic activity exists.

Care of the Patient with a Pacemaker in Flight

1. Check oxygenation and cabin altitude.
2. Treat pain and anxiety.
3. Reduce radio transmissions to a minimum.
4. Secure monitor lead wires and other electrical cables so that they do not swing around.
5. Try to avoid turbulent air.
6. Replace metallic buckles near the pacemaker with other means of securing.

If pacemaker fails, attempt to regain capture by infusion of isoproterenol or adjusting the sensitivity (if a temporary pacemaker). If capture is not returned, treat arrhythmias medically as necessary.

Emergency Landings

A medical emergency as severe as a cardiac arrest or a medical battle to repeatedly correct ventricular tachycardia or congestive failure may necessitate shortening the flight and landing at an airport other than the one planned. Before the decision is made, a number of questions must be asked. All the answers will have some bearing on what the decision should be.

1. How much nearer is the emergency landing airport than the planned destination, judged in flying time?
2. Is there a coronary care unit (or equivalent) in a hospital reasonably near the airport? How far?
3. Is a mobile intensive care unit available to meet the aircraft?
4. Can ground transport and hospital care in the new location be arranged through a "Mayday" radio call within a reasonable period of time?
5. Will care at the emergency location offer any better advanced cardiac life support (ACLS) than the patient is presently receiving?
6. Are there enough suitably experienced personnel presently on board performing ACLS? At least two?
7. Has the care already given depleted any essential supplies (drugs, IV fluids, oxygen, battery power)?
8. Is the aviation environment to be experienced for the rest of the planned flight expected to be enigmatic with regard to any reasonable efficiency of therapy (maneuvers, altitude, turbulence)?
9. Would it improve the patient's care significantly if the aircraft landed sooner so that ACLS could be performed in the stationary aircraft with possible added help from local medical personnel?

The size and capabilities of the aircraft being used will influence some answers. The more suitable the aircraft is as a vehicle in which ACLS can be performed, the more the likelihood that the aircraft will be limited by its runway requirements as to which fields it may use, unless a STOL aircraft such as the Skyvan is being used.

"Mayday." When an emergency landing is contemplated, the pilot must be briefed on the conditions in the cabin. Heed should be taken of his opinions. He will be the one to make the "Mayday" call to air traffic control, identifying the aircraft as a "lifeguard flight" and stating the nature of the emergency. He should be supplied with questions 1 through 4 listed above as a basis for ascertaining the level of care to be expected in the emergency landing environment. The pilot should also be told the answers to questions 6 and 7 by the medical flight attendant, and he should supply the information for the medical attendant to answer question 8. The mobilization of help relative to question 9 would be done by the pilot through A.T.C. or UNICOM. The originally planned receiving hospital and the home base should be informed of the change in mission as soon as possible.

ADJUNCTS TO CARE

Endotracheal Tubes

Check proper placement to ensure tube is in the trachea and not in a mainstem bronchus. Secure the tube to prevent dislodgement during transport. Check cuff pressure. Reduce cuff pressure as cabin altitude is gained. Readjust cuff pressure in level flight. Reinflate cuff on landing if not sealing well.

Tracheostomies

Check that angled adapters are available to connect for oxygenation. Request spare tube and obturator from dispatching hospital or take the same-sized spares if size is known.

Chest Tubes

Chest tubes must not be closed off in flight. Attach a Heimlich valve or finger-cot substitute.

Suction

Check suction apparatus and that the batteries are fully charged and spare batteries are available. Check that suction catheters are with equipment (soft and rigid types). Never prolong suctioning (the patient is not being oxygenated during suctioning). Suction only as catheter is being withdrawn.

Air-Filled Cuffs

Some authorities have recommended using water instead of air to fill the inflatable cuffs of endotracheal tubes or cuffed-tracheostomy tubes. There are as many hazards to this as there are to adjusting the pressure of the air installed. It is not easy to completely fill a cuff without some air being present. Other forces on a water-filled cuff make it more likely to rupture. Modern tubes have a proximal balloon on the air-inlet tube which allows easy testing of the tension in the cuff.

DIABETES MELLITUS

Diabetics must be stabilized before air transfer whenever possible. They should not be transferred less than 5 days after recovering from diabetic coma. Diabetics transported for other illnesses or injuries must also be stabilized and have a plan to meet insulin requirements and nutritional needs worked out with the attending physician. If the diabetes is associated with peripheral vascular disease, special care must be given to prevent constrictions on any blood vessels or muscle masses, and good oxygenation should be provided.

Test tape should be on hand for testing urine for sugar and acetone if the flight is more than 3 hours. Check that there is a supply of 50% dextrose in the flight bag.

For overt hypoglycemia with inability to take oral sugar, give IV dextrose 25 g. Flight preparations should preclude hypoglycemia from occurring, but if there is the slightest possibility that it may occur in a brittle diabetic, the patient should be transported with an IV line. Giving IV dextrose to a patient with tonic contractions that sometimes occur with hypoglycemia can be most difficult without a previously established IV line.

ALCOHOLISM

Alcoholics sometimes get into trouble and have to be transferred home from an overseas appointment or vacation because of their alcoholism and its associated conditions. Requests to evacuate these patients often come before the patient's condition has been controlled to any acceptable degree.

Preflight assessment must pay attention to the recent history and treatment that might indicate that delirium tremens may become overt during transfer. If the patient has some degree of alcoholic intoxication, sedation with hydroxyzine hydrochloride 25 mg IM is recommended before the flight and may be repeated q 2 h prn (up to 4 doses). It would be beneficial to also give thiamine 200 mg IM before the flight, as this may reduce the possibility of convulsions. If the level of consciousness is at all depressed, the patient should be transported with an IV running of 5% dextrose in water KVO. Check whether the patient is also a diabetic or whether this has been ruled out by appropriate investigations. It is of considerable importance to make sure that there is no recent history of head injury or history of convulsions. An anticonvulsant, as well as the thiamine, may need to be given before the transfer.

NEUROLOGIC DISORDERS

Care of patients with neurologic disorders is similar to that for head injuries. The medical flight attendant's concern should be related to and care for:

1. Anxiety (the patient's).
2. Airway patency and oxygenation.
3. Protection of paralyzed and insensitive parts of the body.
4. Convulsions.
5. Unstable body temperature regulation.
6. Sphincter function.
7. Prevention or control of vomiting.
8. Confirm that no pneumoradiologic procedures were recently performed.

PSYCHIATRIC CARE

When requests are received for the transfer of psychiatric patients, a preflight assessment should be performed as for any other medical condition. Special evaluation must be made of the patient's past and current apparent character so that the degree of belligerence or docility to be expected may be judged. A complete record of recent medications and treatment should be made, even though this is sometimes very difficult when the patient has had multiple physicians prescribing multiple drugs.

A medical flight attendant must be constantly aware that psychiatric conditions may be:

1. The manifestation of serious organic disease
2. Produced by drugs (iatrogenic)
3. Play-acting for specific purposes

The first is the reason a preflight assessment should be performed as for any other medical condition. The second is partly the indication for obtaining a complete record of medications used. The third is often difficult to recognize, but an index of suspicion should be maintained in order that unnecessary burdens are not placed on relatives, employees, hospitals, medical personnel, the transporting company, and society in general.

With regard to psychiatric conditions being a manifestation of serious organic disease, one of the more serious mistakes that can be made is the transfer of an intermittently hypoglycemic patient to a psychiatric institution without investigation and treatment of the organic condition. The author is aware of one such transfer being made, but hastens to add that neither he nor the company he was associated with were connected with the transfer.

Legal Responsibilities for Psychiatric Patients

Difficulties can arise regarding who is responsible for giving consent for the transfer and treatment of a psychiatric patient. This must be legally clarified in both the country from which the patient is to be transferred *and* in the country to which he is to be flown. Guardianship accepted in one country may not be accepted in another where religion, customs, and ethics are quite different. The person responsible for the patient should accompany him on the flight, both for legal reasons and for the benefit of the patient so that he is not totally among strangers.

Sedation

Except when the patient is in a catatonic state or where other contraindications exist, sedation should be given to all psychiatric patients before transport. This may need to be done in consultation with the attending physician.

Physical Security

A violent passenger on an aircraft can be a real hazard to the safety of the aircraft and all on board. Should there be any suspicion that the patient has violent tendencies that might not be adequately controlled by sedation, special means of restraint should be available. The straps available on the stretcher, reinforced by judicious bandaging, should usually be sufficient for restraint within the aircraft. Other means of restraint may be needed during ground transport, loading, and unloading.

OBSTETRIC AND GYNECOLOGIC CONDITIONS

There are parts of the world where attitude and religion prevent adequate treatment of women suffering serious complications of childbirth or gynecologic disorders. There are some countries where blood transfusions are not allowed to be given to women. Problems can be prevented by discouraging women advanced in pregnancy from visiting those countries. However, this will not always be possible, and a pregnant woman with a severe hemorrhage may find that her only chance of survival is by air evacuation.

In these cases, it may not be possible to give any IV therapy or blood transfusion until the patient is on board the plane and the doors are closed ready for takeoff. In some cases, pneumatic antishock trousers could be of assistance in maintaining essential circulating volume and in controlling hemorrhage. All intravenous fluids and volume expanders (such as Haemaccel and plasma) and the necessary equipment to administer them must be flown in and remain on the plane. It may be necessary to start an IV line with a large cannula as soon as the patient has been taken on board. There will sometimes be no time for such luxuries as emergency cross-match of blood. Type-specific or type O Rh-negative blood can be lifesaving if it is flown in (assuming the patient's blood type was known beforehand).

Transport of a Patient Near Term

Most airlines are not keen on having an extra passenger arrive on a flight by way of parturition. In practice they do not accept pregnant passengers who are beyond the 35th week of gestation on long flights. Some will accept those who are in the 36th week for a short flight. These rules have limited the number of babies born in the air to such an extent that statistics are limited on whether the aviation environment is inducive to premature labor. The few babies born in the air (reported) suggest that premature labor is not induced, as many women with a tendency to premature labor must have traveled by air in the 35th and 36th weeks of their pregnancies. It is conceivable that a rough flight through excessive turbulence with a seatbelt buckle encroaching on an overlapped lap might physically stimulate labor, but it is doubtful. The author has examined many near-term patients who have been involved in auto accidents (he is sure many of his colleagues also have), and he has rarely noted that trauma induced premature labor. Those reports of labor commencing in the air are often associated with comments that suggest that once labor has commenced in the air, labor progresses more quickly than it would at ground level.

An intentional plan may be drawn to transfer a near-term patient to a specialized facility for her care or for the care of an infant expected to have increased risks as a newborn. The increasing collaboration of obstetricians and pediatricians has led to better recognition of potential problems in the newborn and better identification of those infants that might need neonatal intensive care. With good prenatal care for both the mother and the unborn child (not always synonymous), it is easier to choose the appropriate moment to move the mother to a neonatal intensive care unit. The best means of neonatal transport is still intrauterine, the uterus being better equipped than most modern incubator/respirators designed for neonates.

Risks have to be balanced. Does the mother first have a high-risk infant where there is no neonatal intensive care unit and then have the baby transferred in a specialized, mobile intensive care vehicle or plane to the specialized unit? Or does she allow herself to be transported to a specialized unit near term before labor has commenced, but with the chance that a high-risk neonate may have to be delivered during the transport? Excellent obstetrical care should make the choice obsolete, but situations will still arise where a choice will have to be made. Therefore, it is essential that answers be found to the following questions:

1. What is the nature of the problem expected for the neonate or the mother?
2. What is the expected date of delivery?
3. What complications have occurred during pregnancy?
4. What is the obstetrical history of the mother, including present age and associated medical conditions?
5. Is the receiving hospital and its neonatal intensive care unit willing and ready to receive the mother (and the neonate when delivered)?
6. Is the receiving hospital willing to provide medical flight attendants trained and experienced in obstetrical and neonatal care?
7. Will the hospital provide a neonatal incubator compatible with the aviation environment and the aircraft to be used?
8. What equipment do they have? What is its weight, dimensions, and power source?
9. What ground transportation services are available to meet the aircraft, and how are they equipped and staffed? (It is assumed that the mother-to-be will tolerate the ground transportation from the dispatching hospital to the aircraft or, if not, will be returned to the dispatching hospital for delivery.)

Possibility of Delivery in Flight

Any aeromedical mission which involves the transportation of a female patient with a near-term pregnancy (beyond the 35th week) or a female in the same condition accompanying a patient for whom the mission was planned should be equipped with supplies and equipment to care for both the mother and the neonate in case of delivery in flight.

NEONATAL CARE

Resuscitation of the Newborn

The majority of newborn infants do not require resuscitative measures. Within a few seconds after birth, aspiration of fluids from the mouth and nose with the head down and some stimulation of the skin and feet will elicit bellowing and change of color, thus allaying any fears. However, those newborns that do not respond within 30 seconds should be evaluated quickly for heart rate, neuromuscular tone, and respiratory activity. The latter two are soon obvious. An absent heart sound, a pulse rate below 100 per minute, or inadequate respiratory effort indicates something more should be done. The airway, ventilation, and circulation all require urgent attention. Resuscitative efforts will have less chance of succeeding if the baby is allowed to cool. The fledgling will cool quicker if wet, so he should be dried quickly and kept warm by any means available, possibly including the mother's body.

The Airway

In clearing the airway, the nose is as important as the mouth. Both nostrils should be gently suctioned of any amniotic fluid or blood. If respiratory efforts are inadequate, mouth-to-face breathing should be started immediately. If this is not successful in making the lungs expand, obstruction must be relieved by trying an oropharyngeal airway (if one of the right size is handy—and it should be). If this still does not give a clear airway, intubation will be necessary, followed quickly by mouth-to-tube ventilation until other arrangements can be made to provide oxygen under some pressure.

Even if a full range of respiratory equipment suitable for neonatal care may not be on board, a pocket mask with an oxygen-inlet nipple should certainly be. This may serve as a respirator if used carefully. The mask is best used upside down so that the child's chin is tucked into the nasal groove. The pressure of oxygen delivered can be controlled by occluding the air-inlet port with a finger, watching the thorax rise and removing the finger for expiration.

A special situation should be looked for if the child is in respiratory difficulties. If, as the child was born, the amniotic fluid was clearly stained with meconium, and meconium-stained fluid was aspirated from the nose and mouth, the child should be intubated and the endotracheal tube suctioned as well as possible. Meconium aspiration is a frequent cause of neonatal death or morbidity.

Unless a newborn has congenital problems or is very premature with poorly developed vital centers, correction of the respiratory problems will take care of the cardiovascular status if a heartbeat was present, even though embarrassment was shown by the heart rate being less than 100 per minute. Should there be no heartbeat, or should the rate and force of the heart not be adequate to produce a distal pulse, chest compressions must be instituted—compress the midportion of the sternum ¾ inch, 100 times a minute.

Drug Therapy

In an emergency situation where the newborn requires resuscitative measures but the necessary equipment is not on board, drug therapy will be limited. Epinephrine can be given (if intravenous route not available) by instillation in the intubation tube. The dose should be 0.1 ml per estimated kilogram weight of a 1 : 10,000 solution. Since the newborn rectum absorbs drugs much more quickly than that of someone older, the rectal route might be considered for either epinephrine or atropine (for bradycardia below 80 per minute). The neonatal dose of atropine is 0.03 mg/kg. It used to be believed that the newborn's stomach had the ability to absorb oxygen into the bloodstream. This is not recommended as a means of oxygenation, but a resuscitator might not feel so bad when the stomach has been distended (it is still not desirable). Another drug that might be applicable should it be known that the mother received narcotics within a few hours before birth is naloxone, the narcotic antagonist neonatal dose 0.01 mg/kg.

TRANSPORTING CHILDREN

Children are often more adaptable to medical air transport than adults. It is usually easier to move a child through the various stages because the child can be carried instead of requiring an awkward stretcher. In other ways, children are more difficult to care for. They are more prone to be airsick. They also have more sensitive bladders that respond too easily to excitement. The eustachian tubes of children (in the early years) have an angle and caliber that make them more susceptible to blockage. If the patient is a child, child-sized equipment and doses of drugs should be in the flight bag.

A parent (or both) will usually accompany a child patient. They should be used in the child's care as much as possible, according to the conditions, assuming they themselves are in adequate condition to do so. Occasionally, the parents will be exhausted and overwrought before the flight begins. In such cases it might be wise to prescribe sedation so that they may rest as much as possible during the flight. An upset parent is bound to upset the child patient.

HEMOGLOBIN LEVELS AND ALTITUDE (ANEMIA)

Considering a patient to be transported by air, it has been noted that all tissues need some oxygenation and:

1. The partial pressure of oxygen decreases with altitude.
2. Pulmonary function must be maintained at a level to adequately use any oxygen available.
3. The circulating blood volume must be increased if inadequate, and cardiac efficiency must be assisted if deficient.
4. Electrolyte and metabolic imbalance needs attention.
5. The oxygen-carrying capacity of the blood requires consideration.

The oxygen-carrying capacity of the blood is directly related to the amount of circulating hemoglobin *and* the health of the red blood cells. A diminished level of hemoglobin (anemia) reduces the oxygen-carrying capacity of the blood and therefore the level of tissue oxygenation. A small amount of oxygen is carried in solution in the blood and other body fluids, but not enough to be relied on to provide significant oxygenation of tissues as it is transported in the circulation.

The average healthy adult has approximately 15 g of hemoglobin (Hb) in each 100 ml of blood. One gram of healthy hemoglobin can combine with approximately 1.4 ml of oxygen. The oxygen-carrying capacity of the blood of a normal adult will be (1.4×15) 21 ml $O_2/100$ ml coincidentally, the same numerical value as the percentage of oxygen in the atmosphere. Blood carrying 21 ml $O_2/100$ ml is referred to as being oxygen-saturated 100% (in a patient with 15 g Hb/100 ml).

An anemic patient with less than 15 g Hb must have a smaller oxygen-carrying capacity of the blood even when the blood is fully saturated. Anemia seriously reduces tolerance to a hypoxic environment. The relative tolerance can be considered with an assumption that a patient has fully functioning compensatory mechanisms through increased cardiac output and hyperventilation. An anemia of 7.5 g Hb will have already made demands on those compensatory mechanisms at sea level. The compensatory mechanisms are more efficient when the anemia is chronic in nature than when there has been an acute onset of anemia. With acute blood loss, a tolerable hemoglobin level at sea level—measured after dilution from the correction of volume deficiency—might arbitrarily be nearer to 10 g Hb/100 ml.

A safe level of altitude tolerance without supplementary oxygen should be that altitude at which no discernible signs or symptoms would be expected (in the normal healthy adult this is 6000 feet). From this, an approximation of what the safe levels of altitude will be with various levels of hemoglobin in the blood can be made (Fig. 36). From the same figure the altitude-equivalent of an anemic patient at sea level can be approximated (Table 22).

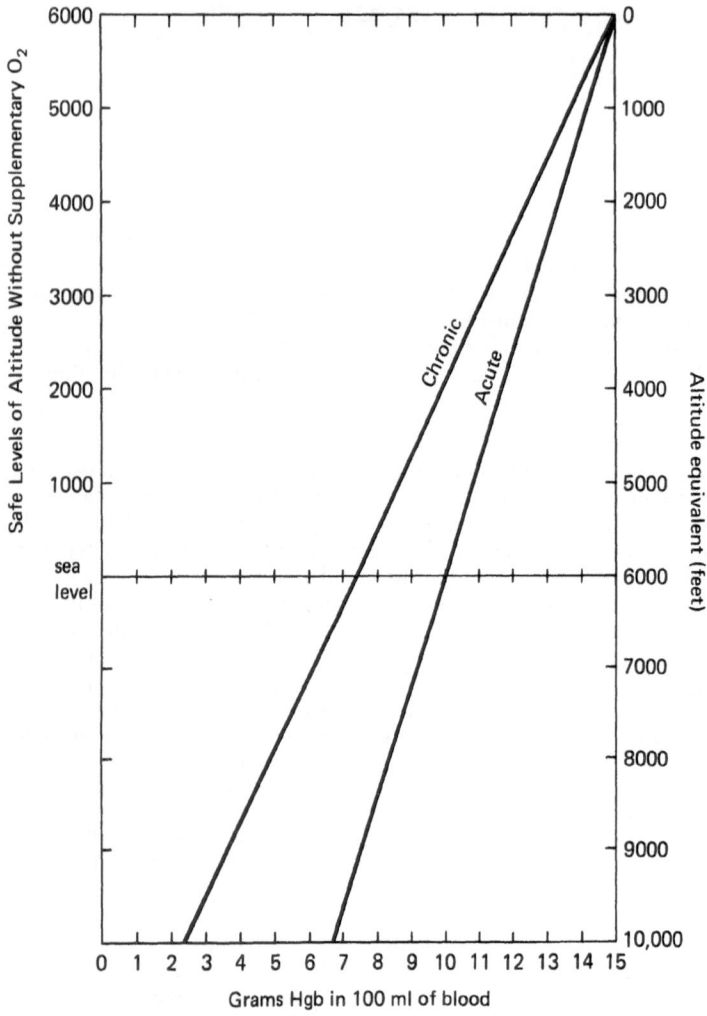

Figure 36.   Safe levels of altitude related to hemoglobin levels.

Differences in Hemoglobin

The foregoing assumptions are calculated with the further assumption
that the hemoglobin has a normal oxygen-carrying capacity. When there
are aberrations in the formula of the molecular constituents of hemoglobin (such as in thalassemia), or when other gases have competed with
oxygen for the hemoglobin (such as when carbon monoxide has combined to form carboxyhemoglobin), the altitude-equivalents are increased and supplementary oxygen is required much sooner for the same
level of hemoglobin. Fetal hemoglobin has more affinity for oxygen, and

Table 22. Patient at Sea Level: Altitude-Equivalent
Related to Hb.

g Hb/100 ml	Altitude-Equivalent (feet)	
	In Acute Anemia	In Chronic Anemia
15	0	0
14	1200	800
13	2400	1500
12	3500	2300
11	4800	3200
10	6000ᵃ	4000
9	7200	4800
8	8400	5600
7	9500	6300ᵃ
6	11000	7200

ᵃ From this table it should be apparent that supplementary oxygen is required at sea level when a patient has only 10 g Hb/100 ml acutely reached, and 7.5 g Hb/100 ml when chronically anemic, if no other reason for supplementary oxygen is present.

the neonate has some advantage in the hypoxic environment. The level of hemoglobin, and whether it is of a chronic nature or of recent origin, is an important item of information to be known at the preflight assessment. In the acute phase, whether dilution has occurred or not must be known.

EMERGENCIES IN THE AIR

An emergency in the air might be defined as any event which presents danger to the patient and/or others on board, and whose onset is unexpected and relatively sudden. This definition can promote an attitude which can ameliorate the consequences of most emergencies. By considering the possible types of emergencies before a flight, any onset of an emergency becomes less unexpected and can have a contingency plan to meet it. Consideration of these contingencies can indicate what equipment might be needed to handle them, and what direct behavior and actions might prevent them from occurring.

Related to Patient

Deterioration of the Patient's Condition
Preflight assessment and ongoing observation during flight should indicate possible future causes for deterioration. Medications, fluids, and

equipment can be chosen which might be needed should deterioration occur. This consideration is the basis for choosing the contents of a medical flight bag.

Some of the major emergencies to be considered are:

1. Hemorrhage
2. Sudden cardiac dysfunction
3. Pulmonary embolus

Hemorrhage and cardiac problems have been previously discussed, and the prevention of air embolus has been considered. *Pulmonary embolus* from thrombosed veins is a serious condition and can be life-threatening.

The history and other information gathered in a preflight evaluation should indicate whether any danger of pulmonary embolus exists. Attention should be paid to whether a patient has had recent surgery, leg or pelvic injuries, or prolonged bedrest without prophylactic physiotherapy. This brings up the point of venous stasis on long flights. It can be discouraged by avoidance of prolonged pressure on the calves and by the encouragement of some movement of the legs.

Sudden deterioration, with elements of shock and respiratory symptoms, could well be due to pulmonary embolus, but pneumothorax must also be considered. Pneumothorax may need to be treated temporarily by needling, and embolus treated for shock and hypotension, with further attention to oxygenation.

Injury to the Patient

Air turbulence and sudden flight maneuvers are likely to be the main causes of injury. Air turbulence cannot always be avoided. Sudden maneuvers should not occur with an experienced pilot, but some may be necessary to suddenly avoid an aerial hazard or to compensate for adverse wind and runway conditions. The jolts from turbulence or sudden maneuvers should not cause injury if sensible precautions are taken. The security of the stretcher frame at its attachment to the cabin floor and the way the patient is secured to the stretcher are obvious points to be watched. Dangers are more likely to come from flying objects in the cabin due to insecure attachment of such things as fire extinguishers and IV bottles. A purposeful inspection of the cabin for loose and potentially detachable items is worthwhile. If injuries are sustained, they must be treated on a first aid basis. Occasionally it may be necessary to suture a laceration if local pressure, steristrip closure, and dressings do not control hemorrhage.

Death of the Patient

Death is not always a medical emergency if it is expected and cannot or should not be prevented. Many aeromedical flights are simply to return a dying patient to his home or to another location of his choice. It *can be* an administrative emergency in that a decision has to be made as to where death occurred. There are more angles to this than might be realized.

Which state, province, canton, or country has jurisdiction to record the death and accept certification? If a particular jurisdiction has interest in the death, the aircraft cannot fly on blithely to its destination which is removed from that jurisdiction. It might have to land in the concerned territory for the authorities to deal with formalities. In most countries, only physicians can pronounce death; the medical flight attendant may not be a physician.

Death may occur over the ocean in international territory. According to the laws of individual countries, there may be differing opinions on the determination of jurisdiction. The place of registration of the aircraft may determine jurisdiction. The aircraft may be registered in one country and may be chartered and manned from another.

Fortunately, there is a certain flexibility present when determining when a patient died. Many certificates and records imply acceptance of the time of pronouncement as being the time of death—*when* determines *where*. In recent years, with the debates on when cerebral death occurs (prompted by the use of life-sustaining equipment in clinically dead patients), the timing of when death occurs has become clouded further.

These facts allow the medical flight attendant some flexibility in legally determining the time of death. At this point, the following rules would logically apply: "On discerning death, radio the nearest local authorities, land in that territory, and take it from there!" or "Record the exact navigational position where death occurred, relate this to the exact time (local or GMT?), and report these facts to the authorities on landing at the destination previously planned. Or, turn back and report to the authorities of where the flight originated." Unfortunately, neither approach is free from administrative problems.

In some cases, complications can occur with unexpected financial and legal implications. An aircraft may land with a deceased patient in one territory, the time and place where death was thought to have occurred having been pinpointed. Both the time and the place can be debated if a physician was not on board (they might be debated even if one was). The territory under the navigational point discerned as being where death occurred may have more interest in the death than recording its happening and its cause. The territory may have explicit laws on death and estate taxes and may claim taxes due, whether the aircraft landed in the territory or not. It may also claim jurisdiction over the distribution of the estate of the deceased. After all, the patient died over its territory.

International maritime laws may sometimes be applicable on international flights, but their logic and precedence will not always help. Ships do not fly over multiple jurisdictions within one country. The sovereignty of states in the U.S. guarantees certain jurisdictions and rights of claim.

It should now be clear how an emergency can be administrative and not only medical or physical. Notification of death must be on a case by case basis, decisions being made by those concerned with the mission and related to its particular circumstances.

Unexpected Death. The unexpected death of a patient in the air requires resuscitative measures by the medical flight attendant using the equipment at his disposal. The pilot should certainly be informed of the occurrence and what is being done in the cabin. With regard to the possibility of an emergency landing, see "Emergency Landings" in the section, Airborne Cardiac Care.

Related to the Attendant

Injury to the Medical Flight Attendant

This certainly should not occur, but it may when the attendant sacrifices some of his own security to attend to some crucial need of the patient. Extra care should be taken, prompted by the realization that it is very much in the patient's interest that the attendant not be injured. An injured attendant is of less or little help to the patient.

When able to be seated, even in calm air, safety belts should be buckled in case of unexpected movements. When caring for the patient in turbulent conditions, shipboard maxims must be followed: Whenever possible—one hand for the ship, one for duties. Sensible bracing against seats and bulkheads may be necessary when both hands are needed. On some occasions, a tie brace may be improvised as used in a ship's galley.

Medical Incapacitation of the Attendant

An attendant with an incapacitating illness should, of course, exclude himself from duty. The most likely medical cause of incapacitation in flight is airsickness. Expected flight conditions should be known, and preventive medication should be taken if necessary. When a decision is made in advance of the flight to take some antiemetic medication, scopolamine dermal patches are possibly the best choice. If the flight is already in progress, meclizine chew tablets might be more appropriate. (See Airsickness later in this part for other hints on how to prevent it.)

Related to the Aircraft

Emergency Landing

The most likely cause for an emergency landing (not at the planned destination or refueling stop) is the development of adverse weather conditions. Inadequate fuel supplies can also be a cause. Fuel might leak (unlikely) or more may be used than expected. Fuel requirements can change during flight according to meteorological conditions. Changes in these conditions can cause a number of changes in altitude, or headwinds can increase in force, both causing increased fuel consumption. The landing may not present much of an emergency for the aircraft if the landing area offers the right facilities, but it may for the patient and the mission.

Malfunction of an engine might necessitate an emergency landing. Most aircraft (except single-engined ones) can fly with an engine shut down, but the performance is diminished. Conditions may be such that it is feasible to continue to the destination; however, if any great distance is to be flown or topographical hazards add undue risk, the aircraft must land elsewhere. An emergency landing due to malfunction in the aircraft will set in motion emergency protocols: firefighting and emergency medical vehicles will be on the emergency airfield, and air traffic control will give priority to the landing. Emergency landing with a malfunctioning undercarriage can be considered a "forced landing."

An unplanned landing may present an emergency for the patient if he has a condition requiring timely definitive care in a hospital environment or is relying on continuous electrical power, oxygen, or other medical supplies that may be disrupted. Efficient communications by radio may best provide for satisfactory care at the unexpected location. What has to be arranged will depend on the expected length of stay and what facilities are available. The medical coordinator of the mission must be immediately briefed on what has happened so that arrangements at the planned destination can be modified and relatives informed. Ambulances waiting for planes that will not arrive as expected do not fit into a cost-effective scenario.

Forced Landings

All forced landings are dangerous. The degree of danger is related to the nature of the terrain to be used, the structural design of the aircraft, and the skill of the pilot. A forced landing implies some notification that one will be necessary. The length of time between notification and landing must be used as efficiently as possible. An attitude must be taken that *excludes* hopelessness. This is vitally important so that every effort is positively directed to meet the inevitable. The manual of operations of each aircraft gives recommendations on land and water forced landings. The pilot must be aware of what those recommendations are and must brief the medical flight attendant.

Actions within the cabin must follow all security arrangements as for a normal landing, *plus* using every extra method that can be thought of to provide physical protection against decelerating forces. These can include using materials such as blankets and coats to cushion and protect the face, neck, and thorax of the patient. How the patient is being secured to the stretcher might be reinforced and considered from the point of view of knowing how best to quickly release the securing devices as soon as possible after the aircraft ceases to move. Note should be made of the location of emergency exits and how they are opened. Flotation devices should be donned, but not inflated, if the landing is to be on water. All preparations for a hasty exit should be made.

Mention might be made of the structural strength of various stretchers and fastenings. Approval of different types by various authorities often focuses on the ability of the stretcher to withstand certain positive or negative G stresses. It is important that a stretcher does not come apart from its fastenings to the floor of the cabin; however, its resistance to collapse with regard to vertical forces *might* be beneficial, but could conceivably be detrimental with regard to the distribution of cushioning forces.

If at all possible, the attendant should be belted in a rear-facing seat for the landing and should follow the instructions of the pilot.

Fire and Fumes

After a forced landing on land, an outbreak of fire may not occur, but actions should be taken as though it will. The patient and the attendant should evacuate the aircraft to a safe distance as soon as is practically possible.

Fire, or any hint of fire, on board an aircraft is an indication for breathing supplementary oxygen from a well-fitting mask. Fire is always accompanied by fumes. The fumes quickly increase in toxicity within the confines of a cabin. Ability to extinguish a fire or take any other remedial action will be quickly lost if fumes are inhaled.

Of the fumes produced by fire, carbon monoxide is the most important one to consider in that it competes with oxygen (unfairly) for attachment to hemoglobin, and the environment soon becomes hypoxic. In healthy subjects at sea level, serious impairment is obvious when the saturation of hemoglobin exceeds 30%. Over 40%, collapse can occur, and most subjects are in coma with a saturation level of 60%. This should stress the importance of immediately using supplementary oxygen, avoiding dilution with cabin air (with a well-fitting mask).

Fire rarely bursts out instantaneously without some prior indication, unless it is the result of an explosion. The three main sources of fire in aircraft are:

1. A malfunctioning engine.
2. Electrical malfunctions
3. The careless handling of burning cigarettes, cigars, or pipes

There are built-in systems to control fire in engines, some of which work automatically and others that are manually operated from the cockpit. Before a fire occurs from an electrical cause, there is almost always an "electrical" smell. Any electrical smell must be thoroughly investigated to determine the source, and the pilot must be informed of its presence. Cigarette-caused fires should not have to be considered on aeromedical flights as all smoking should be banned whether there is a patient on board or not. Apart from the dangers associated with the presence of oxygen, the cabin of an air ambulance should never be allowed to be contaminated with tobacco smoke.

Depressurization

Sudden decompression of the cabin is one of the more serious emergencies in flight. Its seriousness can be judged from the fact that two aviators recently died on a training mission. The depressurization was intentional (termed "dumping"), but supplementary oxygen was not immediately available to the extent expected and disaster ensued.

The physiologic effects depend on the rapidity of decompression. If it is very rapid (less than 10 seconds), the alveoli of the lungs act as semiclosed cavities. The inability to equalize the pressure between the alveoli and the ambient pressure soon enough leaves a pressure differential which can stretch the lung tissue beyond its elastic limits, damaging the lung. The magnitude of the pressure differentials between the lung and that of the depressurized cabin depends on what the cabin/exterior differential is at the time of decompression, as well as the rapidity of pressure loss. The rapidity is determined by the relationship of the volume of the cabin to the size of the defect in the cabin wall. The larger the cabin and the smaller the "hole," the slower the rate of decompression. The reason for small windows and for larger doors opening inward on most aircraft should be apparent.

Except when larger doors "blow" or a large hole occurs in the cabin wall from a missile, most decompressions are not too rapid (usually more than 20 seconds). Depressurization due to failure of the valves or compressors which provide pressurization is relatively slow and can take minutes rather than seconds.

Many aeromedical flights will be in the stratosphere, some as high as

40,000 feet or a few thousand feet more. The seriousness of rapid decompression at high altitudes can be seen in the following table:

Altitude (ft)	Time of Useful Consciousness
40,000	15–20 seconds
35,000	30–40 seconds
30,000	50–60 seconds
25,000	2–5 minutes
20,000	5–10 minutes

These figures are approximations but relate to healthy subjects without the benefit of supplementary oxygen.

If remedial actions are not taken immediately a syndrome of decompression sickness ensues. On aeromedical flights, remedial actions will be taken immediately. They are:

1. Immediate use of supplementary oxygen by all persons on board
2. Rapid loss of altitude to safe levels for unpressurized flight (on aeromedical flights, below 8000 feet)

Most pressurized aircraft have an automatic system which presents oxygen masks when the cabin pressure drops below a specified level for that particular system. Given in terms of relative altitude, it varies between 11,000 and 13,000 feet. A medical flight attendant should know how these systems operate in the particular aircraft being used. The attendant must use the oxygen, be prepared for the plane to make a rapid descent, and ensure the patient is provided oxygen by *mask*.

If decompression was due to a defect larger than a small window, no patching action will be possible. It will be dangerous to approach it in the first few seconds for fear of being ejected from the aircraft. Under fortuitous circumstances, a small window can be partially patched with a rigid object such as a briefcase, reducing the rate of decompression.

After depressurization, when the aircraft is on level flight at a safe altitude, the patient will require considerable attention for vacuum effects in body cavities, for cardiovascular and respiratory stability, and in the form of reassurance.

AIRSICKNESS

Airsickness superimposed upon other medical conditions or injuries can have graver consequences than when it presents in a previously healthy individual. Everything must be done to minimize the chance of it occurring both in the patient and in the medical flight attendant. It can be an incapacitating disorder and can make an attendant totally incapable of performing duties.

Successful prevention depends on knowing the variety of stimuli that provoke motion sickness, of which airsickness is a type. Its name hints that the main cause is motion—and it is. It is *unusual* motion. The vestibular apparatus can tolerate accelerative forces in one direction, and sometimes in two, but problems occur when there are complex directional forces at play. Rotational forces can act in an infinite number of directions, from a vertical pendulum movement to a spinning in any axis as far as the perceptions of the semicircular canals are concerned; accelerating and decelerating forces can be linear vertically, horizontally, or at any angle in between.

It is the complexity rather than the power of the forces that irritates the vestibular apparatus as the bending hairs, moving in the fluid within the canal system, attempt to keep up with orientation in the three dimensions. If one force becomes predominant, it may cancel out the previous confusing stimuli by leaning all the sensitive hairs in the canals, activated by fluid movement, in the same direction opposite to the dominant accelerative force.

Complex motions are the principal cause of airsickness because of the disturbance they cause to the vestibular apparatus. However, other causitive stimuli are of importance because their effects can be mollified. These stimuli are related to the eyes, the gastrointestinal system, ambient cabin temperature, the nose, the psyche, and the brain.

Visual and gastrointestinal stimuli are directly related to the culpable motion. Temperature, smells, and emotions are incidental but play a large part in deciding the severity of symptoms. At times, one or more of them is the provoking cause of the onset of the malady.

Visual Influences

Disorientation can occur when visual stimuli, or lack of them, give interpretations of posture and movement to the brain which are different from those received from the vestibular apparatus. Disorientation is a malady of its own, can be severe, and can have profound psychic effects. It is feared by air crew who have experienced it in any form of severity. It is not knowing which is *up* or *down*. Its severest form is total spatial disorientation. It might be thought that it could be overcome by arbitrarily deciding which is *up* and which is *down*, but this is not possible as that reference is immediately lost. In any case, the *up* chosen is not likely to be the real *up*.

An example of what is involved can be extracted from the consideration of what happens when an aircraft makes a turn. The inner ear feels the beginning of the turn but, if the turn is maintained at an even rate, a neutral condition of the fluid in the semicircular canals is reached (it is not moving) and the inner ear no longer informs the brain that the aircraft is turning. If there are adequate visual references outside of the aircraft (horizon, cloud top, or ground features when at low altitudes), the brain continues the reference to the turn and disorientation does not occur. However, if all the outside visual references are missing, as when in a thick cloud, the senses may give the impression of straight and level flight even though the aircraft is still turning.

Partial disorientation, through cerebral and cerebellar activity, can be an aggravating factor in motion sickness. Its severer form, which can provoke profound psychic changes, is rare because muscle receptors and varying pressures on skin surfaces give some indication of orientation. This is the origin of the expression "Flying through your backside."

Gastrointestinal Influences

The larger the distension of the stomach and the more food or fluid it contains, the larger the force it transmits to its supporting structures. The forces are felt in the epigastrium when forces of movement are more than normal. In the vertical axis, the slower-amplitude vertical motions can stretch the gastric wall, rhythmically provoking retrograde peristalsis with expected results. It is the author's opinion that this is one of the major causes of airsickness concomitant with the vestibular stimuli, and that more attention to gastric comfort can reduce the effects secondary to inner-ear disturbance. As excess salivation is a common early sign of the onset of airsickness, with increased need for swallowing, the stomach is receiving more fluid to aggravate distension. It is possible there is also an increase in gastric secretions.

Temperature Influences

A warm or hot cabin environment is more aggravating to symptoms of airsickness. It could be that olfactory stimuli are sensed more acutely at higher temperatures. A sense of uncomfortable heat is often a symptom of airsickness, and a warmer environment accentuates the feeling.

Olfactory Influences

Certain smells are repulsive and can cause nausea. Olfactory acuity becomes more acute in the early stages of airsickness, and smells normally tolerated become obnoxious. Some patients have reported being able to recognize the smells of such materials as aluminum, plastic, and leather at the same time, and that the confusion of smells was repulsive.

Psychic Influences

It is apparent that in an individual who has previously suffered from any sort of motion sickness, the fear of recurrence is a major contributor to its recurrence. Previous sufferers can be made sick by watching a heaving boat on a movie screen. The placebo effect of anti-motion-sickness medication has been demonstrated. That the psyche plays such an important part in provocation was demonstrated to the author during a preflight assessment when he asked a young patient if he was ever seasick. He immediately turned green and started retching. Words themselves have strong connotations; therefore, the "sick" in airsickness might best be avoided and the condition verbally referred to as "motion malady," or a patient can be simply asked if sea or air travel bothers him.

Influences of Brain Physiology

The term brain physiology is chosen because both the cerebral and the cerebellar elements are involved. It is the confusion of the signals from each element to the other that seems to play some part in the production of the symptoms that we recognize as motion sickness. There is a center in the cerebellum that, when it is extirpated, gives immunity to some symptoms of motion sickness. Some antiemetic agents may act on this center but also act more centrally. Sedation subdues some of the psychic stimuli originating in the cerebrum.

Signs and Symptoms

Premonitory signs of airsickness are often obvious and may be detected in the patient by a medical flight attendant. This will give the attendant an opportunity to modify aggravating stimuli or to treat medically before full-blown symptoms occur. The premonitory signs include increased salivation and swallowing, sweating, pallor, yawning, voluntary hyperventilation, and diminished conversation with lack of attention. The symptoms follow the signs, and an unpleasant epigastric discomfort develops, associated with nausea leading to severe vomiting. A deep psychic depression can acutely occur which sometimes approaches angor animi (the feeling of impending doom). Vomiting can sometimes be accompanied by lack of bladder and bowel control, especially in children who are often more susceptible to motion sickness.

Prevention

In the Patient

Preflight. The tactful history taking, to judge whether the patient is susceptible to motion sickness and to what degree, can provide useful information. If sedation can be combined with an antiemetic action, such medication is desirable. Hydroxyzine hydrochloride is excellent in this respect, given in increments of 25 mg IM up to 75 mg in 4 hours. A large meal or the drinking of excessive amounts of fluid should be avoided within 4 to 6 hours of the commencement of a flight.

In Flight. In the susceptible patient, a supine or semirecumbent position is advisable. A cross-cabin orientation of the stretcher is better than fore and aft. The patient may be advised to keep his eyes closed, not to attempt to read, and not to make sudden movements of the head.

The air of the cabin should not be too stuffy and warm, and a cool ventilator jet may be directed toward the patient's face. Odors might be reduced by avoiding things that produce them. The cabin should be well-aired in advance of boarding if odors are apparent and the outside weather is not inclement. Attention-gaining conversation can divert introspective thoughts which might be dwelling on interpretations of bodily sensations. Physical attention attracts curiosity which can divert the patient's mind from disadvantageous thoughts. This attention may be through the adjustment of belts, pillows, and blankets, or the taking of the pulse and blood pressure.

In the Attendant

Preflight. If an attendant has previously suffered motion sickness of any kind, and a light aircraft is to be used that will be spending much of the flight in the weather altitudes, some prophylactic medication might be advisable. The one less likely to cause undue drowsiness or other side effects is scopolamine, when used in tiny doses as provided by its release from a dermal disk placed behind the ear. It is marketed in the U.S. as Transderm-V and can give some protection for many hours. A disk should be placed on the hairless skin behind an ear approximately 2 hours before the flight. The same advice regarding eating and drinking before a flight is applicable to attendants as well as patients.

In Flight. The concentration required by duties should exclude the psychic elements that might provoke motion sickness. Frequent physical movement deflects the senses from those that might be confused (as they are in disorientation) and those that might pay excessive attention to gastrointestinal stimuli. In two words—"Be busy." However, sudden head movements should be avoided. Frequent change of visual sights from outside the cabin to inside objects or instruments requiring narrow focus should also be avoided. The ventilation of the cabin should be attended to. Should the premonitory symptoms be recognized and if preflight antiemetic medication was not taken, a chew tablet of meclizine (Bonine) 25 mg may abort the onset.

Treatment of Established Airsickness

In the patient, protection of the airway is paramount. Antiemetic medication should be given if not already received. If it has been received before the flight, an antiemetic of a different type may be tried or the original medication repeated if dosages allow. A patient with some fragility of fluid balance may need IV fluid replacement. The fluid loss from excess vomiting can itself sustain the feeling of nausea and provoke more vomiting.

4

APPENDICES

APPENDICES

INTERNATIONAL MISSIONS

Time Zones

When a mission is to be flown from one time zone to another, it is important that the time difference be established early on in the planning of the mission. All times recorded must note where they relate to. A time-zone map of the world gives some indication what the time differences will be between various locations, but nations alter times twice a year, not always on the same day worldwide. During a preflight assessment, the time difference can be established and, if it is early Spring or Fall, inquiry should be made as to whether the clocks will change during the next few days.

Interesting situations can arise from these time differences, especially when the date line is crossed. One baby arrived in Hong Kong the day before his birthday! When missions are to cross the date line, the day of the week should always be related to the date so that coordinators at both ends of the mission are talking about the same day. The local time of where the patient is picked up should be used with regard to when to give treatments and medications. This time schedule should be kept to until the patient has arrived at the receiving facility.

Climate

The climate at both ends of a mission and at any stopovers is important with regard to supplies to promote thermal comfort for the patient and his attendant. For the patient, light thermal blankets are better than thick ones, and nylon should be avoided if possible to reduce static electricity. An aircraft cabin may get quite cold even in tropical climes at altitude should the heating system be deficient. The author has been on an airstrip at the equator on the lower slopes of Mount Kenya where the ground temperature was below 40°F in the morning. Therefore, blankets should always be carried.

For the attendant, thermal comfort is best achieved by a choice of clothing which can provide insulation without bulk and excessive weight. The character of the underclothes should be adapted rather than adding outer garments. Leaving a cloudy, temperate climate, the need for sunglasses, sunscreen creams, and cold fluids may not be too apparent. However, flying often carries the attendant into very bright sunlight at moderate altitudes where sunglasses are needed to make accurate observations and readings. Leaving a tropical zone for colder climes, the need for gloves to protect the hands from the metal on a stretcher may be forgotten, as may the need for warm beverages.

An ill or injured patient may be much more sensitive to extremes in climate. The neonate or small infant is especially sensitive to low temperatures and must be carefully protected from hypothermia.

Language

An interpreter may often be required; if so, he should have some knowledge of medical terminology, if possible. This can prevent some embarrassing misinterpretations. (There is a sameness about some medical terms in a variety of languages, which is of some help.) Accuracy of information is sometimes vitally important, and misinterpretation could lead to disaster. Any aid that might increase the accuracy should be carried and used. Many polyglots covering the medical terms and phrases in many languages are available and make a useful addition to any flight bag. Pointing to parts of the body or the use of diagrams may also clarify points.

It should be noted that interpreters are sometimes required to understand someone who supposedly speaks the same language. Dialect and colloquial use of words can cause confusion. For example, some Englishmen cannot understand Australians, and some Englishmen cannot be understood by anyone! A West-Country man may say "Tintontoym"—this means "It isn't on time." An Australian saying "Owk eye" means "Yes."

A medical flight attendant may have to suffer some embarrassment by exposing his ignorance when attempting to interpret a medical fact. Embarrassment, however, is preferable to lack of accurate information.

Ethics and Culture

An example of how this may affect the accomplishment of a mission was described earlier under Obstetric and Gynecologic Conditions. The ability to use services at an airport, in some countries, may depend to a considerable extent on whether some bribe or reward is offered. As objectionable as this may seem to those unused to this behavior, it may need to be resorted to for the safety and benefit of the patient. A lecture on Western morality might be a waste of time and counterproductive in some cases where some essential service or supply is needed. Objection to corruption may sometimes be mollified by considering the dire needs of those requiring bribes. Recognition of cultural differences is important to ensure a medical flight attendant always appears courteous and grateful to the officials and the medical personnel he will meet in foreign countries. A wrong impression can present problems that will reflect on the ability to do the best for the patient.

Political Systems

The level and nature of security protocols and the strictness with which they are enforced depend on the political system of the country visited. Previous knowledge of what those protocols are is essential on some missions. For example, on a mission flown from some countries to Russia (assuming clearance has been obtained for an aircraft to enter Russian territory), the aircraft must land at particular airports near the border for a Russian pilot or navigator to join the crew for the flight to the pickup point and return. Since there must be room for the Russian flight officer to be on board for this part of the misison, this might place further limits on the number of persons able to be on board on the outbound leg.

The strictness given to entrance and exit permits, health regulations, and customs and excise inspections depends on the host country's relationship to that country from which the aircraft originated, the country of registration of the aircraft being used, and the nationality (and sometimes the religion) of the flight crew (cockpit and medical) and the patient. There will be times when an aircraft will have to be chartered from some other country and a flight crew chosen having a particular nationality or religion (or *not* having a particular nationality or religion) to accomplish the mission between certain points.

Flight Plan Clearances

Some air charter companies, including some air ambulance units, may have prior clearance to enter particular countries. This can save a lot of time when a mission is requested on an emergency basis.

Whenever an aircraft flies to another country, it must have clearance to land or enter the territory *before* the mission is flown. From one country to another friendly country, when prior international agreements have been made, permission may be easily obtained at the time the pilot files his flight plan. Otherwise, permission may be difficult to obtain and involve consular- and embassy-level communications of extended length and complexity. A mission cannot be flown with the hope permission will be granted in the air or on landing. An aircraft may be impounded, grounded, and put out of use for many weeks. The crew may languish in a jail without any benefit to the patient who had requested transfer. It is hoped that international agreements will be on a wider scale in the future and give more urgent priority to missions of mercy. The turmoil present in many parts of the world does not make this a likely possibility.

Use of Military Installations

Whereas some political situations can add problematic complexities to international medical missions, it must be pointed out that many countries in the world desire to be of assistance to foreign nationals requiring medical air evacuation. This may extend to offering the use of airfields that are usually reserved for military or official government aircraft. The Kenyan government only recently gave permission for the Flying Doctors of Africa to use a government airfield in Nanyuki, which was of great benefit to a patient being transferred to Nairobi by air.

When military airfields are used, previous permission and arrangements having been certified, an amount of caution is required on landing. No one on board should attempt to disembark until an official who is aware of the legality of the landing has come to the plane and cleared the exit. There is a high possibility the plane will be surrounded by armed sentries, some of whom may not have been briefed on the aircraft's arrival. A premature exit may thus prompt a dangerous welcome.

Entry Requirements

A valid passport is not always enough to grant entrance into a country should a medical flight attendant have to leave the aircraft and proceed to where the patient is located. In some places it may not even be enough to leave the aircraft and proceed into the airport terminal or buildings. Documents may be necessary in the form of an official letter from a recognized representative of the country who has the proper authority to issue such a document. The document may be in the form of a valid visa—stamped, dated, and signed.

New visas often take many weeks to acquire. Multiple-entry visas are useful when there is a likelihood a medical flight attendant will be making more than one trip to the same country. Emergency visas can be difficult to obtain, but many consulates can be extremely helpful. Being prepared ahead of time in case an emergency application for a visa is necessary can help and can speed the process. Duplicate passport photographs should always be kept with the passport, along with the birth certificate and a copy of a medical or nursing license. When the visa is actually applied for, a written statement of who the patient is, his medical condition and problems necessitating the evacuation, and the name of the hospital he is in and under whose medical care will most likely be required. The more complete *written* information *appears*, and the more documents that can be offered with the application, the quicker and easier a decision *might* be arrived at and a visa issued.

Customs and Excise

On entering a foreign country, three authorities are concerned with the entrance: the immigration officer, the health officer, and the officer responsible for preventing the entry of contraband and collecting duty on certain imported items. The duties of the three may be combined in one or two individuals or shared between 20 or 30 with varying levels of authority.

A medical flight attendant will be carrying medical equipment and a flight bag containing instruments, drugs, and medicaments. These require inspection or disclosure for the information of the customs officer. If a medical flight bag is clearly marked as such with appropriate emblems, and an inventory list can be presented describing all the contents in detail, there will rarely be other than a cursory inspection and no difficulty should be experienced clearing the inspection station. Without an inventory list, it may be impossible to completely describe the contents and, in all probability, a more thorough inspection may ensue. For security reasons, the attendant must always be present to observe any inspection procedures. No drugs should be missing from the inventory list; otherwise, serious charge of attempting to smuggle in illicit drugs might be made, with serious consequences for the attendant and delay in reaching the patient.

Health Regulations

To gain entry into some countries, evidence must be presented to show that certain immunizations are current. Smallpox used to be the most important vaccination required, but as it has *almost* been eradicated, most countries have relaxed their regulations requiring current vaccination (within 3 years) for entrance. There is still some risk, though slight, in a few countries, and health officers still maintain vigilance on the chance new cases will surface. It is only 5 or 6 years ago that there were infective cases in Ethiopia. The disease is most likely to be found in areas where travelers rarely visit. Medical attendants who may travel to the interior of Africa, South America, or tropical areas of Asia should consider revaccination every 3 to 5 years.

The most serious diseases that warrant continued vigilance and immunization programs to prevent contraction and spread are yellow fever and polio. The latter has not been given the attention it deserves by some of the health authorities in the countries where it has been found, and few if any demand proof of polio immunization for entrance. Many countries still require proof of satisfactory yellow fever immunization before entrance. These are not only countries where the disease has been known to exist but others that have never had cases of the disease but see their climate, topography, and insect poulation as potentially providing the setting for the entrance and spread of the disease. Yellow fever is still endemic in Central Africa and in Central and South America as far down as 20° south of the equator. Fortunately, the vaccine that gives satisfactory immunization against yellow fever is effective for 10 years after one injection. A medical flight attendant on a mission to a country requiring yellow fever immunization for entrance or where it is known to be endemic should surely make that immunization a top priority in any vaccination program.

Requests for medical transfer of patients with active endemic diseases such as plague, smallpox, or yellow fever must be refused. The ramifications of transferring a patient with an infective disease that could place numerous persons or even whole populations at risk are far too serious. Such a request might be humanely answered by an offer to arrange for a specialist in the disease (who is himself immunized against it) to be flown to the patient if such a specialist is not available in that country.

International Health Regulations (IHR)

IHR are published by the World Health Organization (W.H.O.), the headquarters of which is in Geneva. The regulations are designed to control the spread of diseases, and they concern themselves with immunizational procedures, quarantine methods, and the prevention of transmission of diseases and disease vectors (insects, rodents, and infected humans and other animals). The IHR consolidate the health regulations issued by many countries. Those of some countries differ in some respects and may be more stringent than others according to the problems and risks perceived. The regulations have great importance in this age of long-distance international travel involving millions of people.

The ability of the W.H.O. to modify the regulations and recommendations depends on the quality and frequency of reports from individual member nations. From these reports, the W.H.O. publishes lists of designated sanitary airports and those free from the risk of malarial transmission. To be designated a sanitary airport, it must have certain medical facilities capable of public health studies as well as supervised quarantine areas. It must also be free from disease vectors within specified distances of the airport terminal. The W.H.O. also publishes a weekly epidemiological record for subscribers in English and French. It also publishes a yearly updated "Vaccination Certificate Requirements for International Travel."

Aircraft General Declaration of Health

Health authorities in any foreign country may require a formal completion of the health part of the Aircraft General Declaration. This would involve the pilot notifying the authorities of any person on board suffering from an illness other than airsickness. The medical flight attendant should assist the pilot in making his report, indicating to the authorities that the patient is not a danger to others from the point of view of infectivity. Delays may be prevented by notifying the authorities in advance by radio that an ill or injured patient is on board. Radioing details of the patient's condition may hasten evaluation on landing and expedite patient care at the airport.

Disinsection and Disinfestation

IHR stipulate which procedures are approved for disinsection and disinfestation of aircraft on international flights. Insects and rodents can gain entrance into an aircraft: into the cabin, storage holds, or undercarriage bays. Cockroaches are possibly the most resourceful insects; fortunately, they are not too harmful. Their extinction in an aircraft is often a measure of how successful procedures have been to disinsect the aircraft. The mosquito is a vector of a number of diseases. Aircraft that travel to mosquito-infested areas must take precautions to make sure mosquitoes are not carried into or out of a country. To ensure this, certain spraying techniques are specified by the IHR.

The choice of chemicals and methods must take into account the insects' hiding places, and that only chemicals be used which present no health hazard and which will not structurally damage the aircraft or its seals. In light aircraft, the approved method of disinsection is the full discharge of an aerosol can of insecticide providing 1 g per 100 cubic feet of cabin volume. The correct number of cans must be used (depending on estimated cabin volume), and the empty cans must be saved as supporting evidence that disinsection was carried out. The "blocks away" method is when the spray is discharged after all are on board and just before takeoff. When traveling to a country that requires a report of disinsection, the spray should be used at the last airport before arrival in that country. The pilot must have a certificate of disinsection signed by an airport health official. The certificate will be part of the health declaration that might be requested by the health officer at the destination.

At smaller airports where control of rodents may be lax or nonexistent, the possibility of rats entering the aircraft must be kept in mind, and doors should not be left open unattended and unobserved. Not only can rats present a hazard as disease vectors (especially for plague), they can also chew and damage parts of the aircraft that may be vital to its safe operation.

Malarial Areas

Malaria is far from being eradicated. The hope in D.D.T., which proved itself able to disinsect large areas, was dashed when it was learned that the chemical enters the animal-plant food cycle and that many insects became resistant to it.

Malaria is present in many areas of the world. As different types of malaria are prevalent in different areas, and prophylaxis recommendations vary from territory to territory, one method of prophylaxis cannot be generally recommended. A medical flight attendant who will be exposed to mosquitoes in a malarial area must take whatever prophylactic medication is recommended for that territory. Ideally, the medicine should be started 1 or 2 weeks before journeying to the area, but this will rarely be practical on evacuation missions. Therefore, medication should be taken as soon as the necessity is apparent. It must also be continued for 6 weeks after returning from the area.

As the attendant is usually not fully protected at the time of arrival in a malarial area, precautions should be taken to minimize the chance of being bitten by mosquitoes. Knees should not be bare, long sleeves should be worn, and the clothing and exposed skin should be regularly sprayed with insect repellent. On short stays of a few hours, these precautions may seem excessive. The chances of being bitten by a malaria-carrying mosquito may be very small, but the author is aware of a tragic ending for someone who was not fully protected. The wife of his chief flew from England to join her husband in South Africa. The plane made a stop for some hours in a West African territory. It was assumed that she had been bitten by a malaria-carrying mosquito during the stopover and tragically contracted a malignant form of the disease from which she died.

Other Endemic Diseases

Malaria, yellow fever, and smallpox have been discussed in detail earlier. Polio was briefly mentioned.

Poliomyelitis

Polio can strike in almost any country where enough members of the population are not fully immunized against it. Because it is one of the easiest diseases to immunize against and was so successfully reduced in frequency of appearance in the 1950s and 1960s, it has not retained the respect and concern of the general public or younger physicians and nurses who did not witness its terrible effects. Laxity has developed in the attitude toward poliomyelitis. It is, however, still sporadically occurring in many countries. Anyone who travels widely or medical flight attendants who have never suffered from polio and have not been reimmunized with a booster for the last 10 years should receive a booster.

Plague

Because the author witnessed an outbreak of respiratory plague in an East African territory less than 2 years ago, he has a fearful respect for the disease. The risks of a short-term visitor catching the disease are remote if a reasonable degree of hygiene is maintained and rat-infested areas are avoided.

The better-known type of the disease is one which has a longer natural history and has historical references, bubonic plague. This is less serious than the respiratory type which has a rapid onset and can kill within a few days. In the outbreak mentioned, no persons of European origin contracted the disease. It was related to an excessive infestation with rats in a native quarter (the incubation period is 6 days). What is troublesome about plague is that it can be spread by an infected person directly to others without a vector being required. In this respect it is like smallpox and hepatitis. Smallpox, plague, and cholera can also be spread by contamination of objects or surfaces.

Cholera
For those in reasonable health and in a good state of nutrition, cholera is a nuisance disease that can be treated relatively easily in the right surroundings. Immunization against the disease is not very effective. Most countries do not now require proof of immunization before entry. Preventing the spread of the disease is possibly more important than the treatment protocols (unless one is the patient).

Typhus
Like plague, it is a danger where hygiene is deficient and rodents abound. It is unlikely to be contracted by a short-term visitor unless on a mission to the interior of a country under rough circumstances.

Typhoid
Those who have always lived in an ultrahygienic society where plastic wrappings keep fingers and flies off food and sterilization of food and flavor is common have an increased susceptibility to the typhoid bacillus and its colleagues, paratyphoid A and B. New travelers to distant and dirty (relatively) places must take more precautions with regard to what is eaten or imbibed. Gastrointestinal problems do not necessarily mean the typhoid family is active; it is more likely an *Escherichia coli* novel to the particular gut. Unless a medical flight attendant is experienced in choosing native foods and beverages, he would be wise to avoid them on a short-term mission and take along nourishment he can rely on.

Amebic Dysentery
Amebic dysentery is a more serious condition than the bacterial enteric diseases. If it is not recognized and treated early, infection can spread to the liver and sometimes to the lungs. The same precautions of hygiene taken to avoid the other enteric diseases will prevent infection from the ameba. They are more important, in the case of amebic dysentery, as there is no effective method of immunizing against it.

Infectious Hepatitis
Although this disease is common in the United States, there seems to be some evidence that it can be contracted more easily in tropical and subtropical countries, possibly because of the larger number of insects that might assist the fecal-oral contamination route. Cups and eating utensils should not be shared with casual friends.

Schistosomiasis
When visiting an exotic or out-of-the-way place abroad, it is often tempting to take a relaxing swim in a stream, pond, or lake. However, beware of schistosomes. Careful inquiry should be made of knowledgeable locals as to whether it is safe to enter the water.

Immunization Requirements

There are two types of requirements: one to meet the regulations for entry into a particular country, and one related to the personal health needs of the individual. Immunizations required for entry have been addressed. Those to be considered for personal protection depend very much on where an individual might travel in the near future. Some immunizations give protection for a limited length of time and are soon out of date. It also depends on the previous immunizational history and whether conditions exist, such as allergies or skin diseases, that would modify any immunization program.

It is hard to find any consensus of opinion for any particular circumstance, and the extent of immunizational advice can vary from recommending every vaccine known to man to the minimum required for entry. When risks are very slight but are nevertheless present, it is hard to make compromises. Some immunization procedures carry their own risks. What is to be used must be a joint decision of the physician and patient, the patient being made aware of the risks. Too many immunizations seem to fatigue the immunological system of the body, so that some procedures could become counterproductive. Protection thought to have been obtained from vaccination procedures should never be taken for granted and never used as an excuse for relaxing hygienic standards and sensible behavior.

TRANSFER OF PATIENTS BY SCHEDULED COMMERCIAL AIRLINES

All airlines have different degrees of willingness or reluctance to transport ill or injured patients on scheduled flights. The reluctance is understandable, as a considerable amount of organizational and logistical work is involved to provide space for the patient, special stretchers and other equipment, and special services for embarking and disembarking. The adaptable stretcher, its attaching frame, and the necessary hardware and tools necessary to make the installation may not be available at the airport of origin and may need to be flown in from some other location. It is not cost-effective to have all such equipment at every airport the airline uses. At most airports, a variety of wheelchairs and other invalid aids will be found, but some organization is required for them to be at a particular location at a specific time.

There is often the danger, in the minds of airline officials, that the condition of a patient may deteriorate in flight or he may die, or that the flying experience will aggravate illness or injury. The appearance, smell, or sound of certain patients may be disturbing to other passengers. Psychiatric patients may be a danger to the crew, passengers, and the aircraft itself. All these considerations necessitate careful examination by the airlines' medical departments of any request to transport a patient.

If a reservations department of an airline is requested to reserve space for transport of a patient, it will refer the request to the airline's medical department and provide the requesting physician with a medical certificate form for completion and signature. It should be noted that when the form is signed, it is certifying that the patient is not *infectious* and will not cause *distress, inconvenience,* or *embarrassment* to other passengers. It also certifies that the patient is medically fit to undertake the journey. These factors should be in mind during the preflight assessment. Each request will be judged on its merit from either a purely medical angle or possibly from a humanitarian point of view if the flight will make the difference as to whether the patient lives or dies. Certain types of cases will almost certainly be rejected for airline transfer, though a few exceptions occur.

Cases Unacceptable to Commercial Airlines

1. Infectious, contagious, and all communicable diseases.
2. Facial sinus or middle-ear disease, and when there has been recent surgery on the ear (especially stapedectomy).
3. Those who have received radiologic and other diagnostic studies which involved the introduction of air into body cavities or tissue planes (within 7 days).
4. Pregnancy beyond the end of the 35th week (maybe 36th week for short flights).
5. Severe anemia.
6. Recent abdominal surgery (within 10 days).
7. Recent chest or cranial surgery (within 20 days).
8. Myocardial infarction (within 6 weeks).
9. Peptic or intestinal disease with history of hemorrhage within 3 weeks.
10. Severe hypertension and congestive heart failure.
11. Repulsive-looking skin lesions.
12. Some mental cases with violent history.

The Stretcher and Loading

Just as every patient occupying a hospital bed is not bedridden, every stretcher patient is not incapacitated to the degree of not being able to leave the stretcher for a few minutes to be moved by wheelchair. The stretcher frames and stretcher, specially designed for use in commercial airliners (and approved by various authorities), have to be correctly fitted into the aircraft *before* the arrival of the patient. To load the patient, a breakaway stretcher may need to be carried on board, then the patient transferred to the airline stretcher. Large as the doors of the bigger airliners may seem, many present one problem or another making the turn into the long axis of the cabin. A carry-on stretcher may need to be lifted at a height to clear seat tops and other obstructions. If the patient is able to be transferred into a wheelchair for the loading, some loading problems can be avoided. However, an ordinary wheelchair with armrests is too wide to be wheeled down most airliner aisles. A specially designed wheelchair that is quite narrow and has no projecting armrests will be needed.

Oxygen

The final responsibility for the use of oxygen on board rests with the commander of the flight, the pilot. This is by inference from aviation regulations. Because of this, most airlines insist that all oxygen to be used by a patient on a flight be supplied by the airline. Permission will occasionally be granted for special oxygen equipment to be provided by those caring for the patient, but it is usually required that an official of the airline inspect what is to be used.

Arranging Transport by Scheduled Airline

Those arranging the medical transfer by scheduled airliner also have a considerable amount of organizational work to do before a flight. A checklist is useful so that important details are not overlooked:

1. Preflight assessment of the patient, and collection of pertinent medical records.
2. Complete standard airline medical certificate.
3. Identify airports that can be used (and alternates), and know the facilities there for embarkation and disembarkation.
4. Identify airline(s) and current route schedules.
5. Check if any seats are available on most convenient flight.
6. Liaison with medical department of airline as to whether patient might be accepted and, if so, tariffs to be charged.
7. Seat plan to indicate seats assigned for stretcher area (note nearness to entrance, exits, and toilets).
8. Arrangements for oxygen supply.
9. Will airline provide necessary stretchers, wheelchairs? Will they allow equipment to be used, supplied, and chosen by the medical flight attendant?
10. Equipment to be carried by medical flight attendant. Request prior authority to take equipment and personal luggage into the cabin. (Gate supervisors may attempt to prevent even the flight bag containing necessary drugs and equipment from being taken into the cabin, and they may insist on it being checked in.) Portable, wheeled luggage carrier. Minimal personal luggage.
11. Any nutritional needs in flight not available from the airline?
12. Ground ambulance arrangements.
13. Passport, visa, and health regulations.
14. Reservations for overnight stays by medical flight attendant.
15. Cash requirements or payment arrangements for expenses on mission.
16. Contingency plans in case of delays, unexpected stopovers, or last-minute change of decision to transfer.

The pilot will already have been briefed that a stretcher patient might be on board. The medical flight attendant should introduce himself to the captain upon boarding. He should be briefed on the important aspects of the patient's condition. The flight deck crew will radio ahead in time to confirm that the ground ambulance will be waiting in the correct area of the airport. With a patient on board and the flight designated "lifeguard," some priority may be given to the flight should holding patterns delay landing.

Airline cabin attendants can be helpful with regard to the provision of minor needs such as wipes, towels, and ice. They can also help with food items and substitutes from the main meal. They cannot be expected to provide any nursing services. As one of their main duties is the handling of food, they must never be asked to assist in carrying or emptying bedpans or urinals.

Both the cabin crew and the flight deck crew often welcome the presence of medical personnel with medications and diagnostic equipment, especially on long oceanic flights. It removes a burden from them, to some extent, should a medical emergency occur among the passengers or the crew.

As an example of the policies of international airlines based in the United States, the following is quoted from a communication with the Corporate Medical Director of Pan American World Airways.

> Government (FAA) approved stretchers are the only ones permitted, and they are supplied by the company. Wheelchairs are available at all airports to assist passengers. Oxygen equipment is supplied only by the airline; passengers are not by law permitted to carry their own oxygen equipment aboard the aircraft. Our oxygen bottles are 300 liter capacity with a choice of two different oxygen rates of flow—two liters per minute for approximately 150 minutes, or four liters per minute for approximately 75 minutes. Oxygen requirements for a multi-sector flight can be arranged and are planned for a resupply at enroute stations thereby minimizing the use of on-board storage space. Each oxygen bottle costs $85.00 in advance, non-refundable. Special arrangements can be made for the use of 100 cu. ft. oxygen bottles and in such cases the seat adjacent to the passenger requiring the oxygen is blocked off for bottle storage.
>
> Any other equipment required for use by the passenger, such as suction apparatus, bedpan, etc. must be supplied by the passenger. Only respirators which will operate on 115 volts and 60 cycles can be connected to the aircraft electrical current.

Documentation Required by Airlines Before Transporting an Incapacitated Passenger

Most passenger-carrying airlines are members of the International Air Transport Association. When arranging for an ill, injured, or physically incapacitated passenger to be transported, use forms internationally recommended by I.A.T.A. Some airlines modify the forms to suit their own requirements. The forms are available at the reservation counters or may be obtained from the medical departments of the airlines. The print on the forms is very small, so a reduction for the purpose of showing copies in this text would make them unreadable. They may be obtained from the airlines or by writing to the International Air Transport Association, 1000 Sherbrooke Street West, Montreal, Quebec, Canada H3A 2R4, or 26, chemin de Joinville, 1216 Cointrin, Geneva, Switzerland.

I.A.T.A. also publishes a medical manual and a number of useful booklets including "Incapacitated Passengers Physicians Guide" ($2.00 US) and "Incapacitated Passengers Handling Guide" ($2.50 US) for airline and travel agency staff.

The forms (known as Medif forms) are in two parts. Part one must be signed by the patient or the patient's representative and authorizes a physician (named) to provide the necessary medical information. It also provides information essential to the planning of the transport, including the following:

1. Proposed itinerary
2. Nature of incapacitation
3. Whether a stretcher is required on board
4. Name and qualifications of the medical attendant
5. Whether a wheelchair is required and its type
6. Ambulance arrangements
7. Other ground arrangements at departure, connecting, and arrival points
8. In-flight needs: equipment, special seats, extra seats, meals
9. Whether the passenger has a Fremec card (a card available to physically incapacitated passengers who travel frequently)

When the patient or his representative signs part one, agreement is made to accept responsibility for any change in medical condition that might occur from being transported by air and for any financial costs incurred.

Part two of the Medif form is to be completed by the physician responsible for the patient. The information the physician must supply includes the following:

1. Details of the illness or injury, including the dates of the first symptoms or accident and the date the relevant diagnosis was made
2. Prognosis for the journey
3. Whether any contagious or communicable disease
4. Whether the patient would be in any way offensive to other passengers because of smell, noise, or appearance
5. Whether the patient can use a normal aircraft seat with the seat back in the upright position
6. Whether the patient can take care of any of his own needs such as visiting the toilet and eating the meals normally provided
7. Whether the arrangements for an attendant (as outlined in part one of the form) are satisfactory to the responsible physician
8. Oxygen requirements
9. Medications and special equipment, such as IVs or respirator, required during transport on the ground and in flight

10. Arrangements for hospitalization at arrival point or for overnight stay at a connecting point
11. Any other information useful to the airline for the care of the patient
12. Details of other arrangements made by the attending physician

All the information on both parts of the Medif form must be available to the medical flight attendant accompanying the patient.

THE FUTURE OF AIR AMBULANCING

The Present State of the Art

In 1982, the quality of care and safety for patients being transported by air in the United States is not consistently satisfactory. Although there has been a steady increase in the number of aeromedical flights in recent years, air ambulancing is still at the stage of development (in civilian practice) at which ground ambulancing was 12 or 14 years ago. In those days, there were few ground ambulance units that gave adequate prehospital care and transport, judging by present-day standards. It took a tardy explosion of public and professional awareness to give the necessary attention and thought that would dramatically improve the standards of training, equipment, and organization. The development of emergency medicine, emergency nursing, and critical care; the supervision of the training and proficiency of ambulance personnel; and the regulation of vehicles and their equipment have proceeded concomitantly. Citizens have reaped many benefits now taken for granted.

The quality of medical care in the air, however, cannot be taken for granted everywhere in the United States. There are some air ambulance companies that have elevated their service and proficiency to a level that should be an example for others. However, there are others that purport to be air ambulance operators that in no way meet proficiency standards.

Many well-meaning attempts have been made, on a federal level, to regulate air ambulances. They have failed for a number of reasons, not all unjustified. Some states have adopted regulations. The Federal Department of Transportation has collaborated with a committee of the American Medical Association to publish guidelines for the operation of air ambulances. It is hoped these guidelines will draw attention of physicians to the need for medical control in the field.

Standards can be set by widespread mutual agreement, example, and the inherent wish to improve what can be improved. The means to do so only need exposing. Such a way of improving standards can be faster, less painful, less expensive, and more fruitful than by bureaucratic regulation. As was the case of the movement that produced great improvements in ground ambulancing, publicity and enthusiasm should be all that is required to prompt the elevation of aeromedical care to a proficient level. It is the hope of the author that parts of this book will serve

some purpose toward fanning enthusiasm for aeromedical care as a vital
dimension of the emergency medical services.

The Need

Individuals becoming ill or injured many miles from their homes (sometimes in foreign lands) are often more appropriately transported by air.
Occasionally, there is no alternate means of medical transport. Tertiary
medical care centers, with specialized services not available elsewhere
within land range, have prompted more aeromedical transfers. Many
more aeromedical flights would be made but for the cost being prohibi-
tive for the majority of persons. The underutilization of dedicated air
ambulances further increases the cost to the ones who do use them.

Insurance

The answer to making medical air evacuation more accessible to those
who could benefit from the service would seem to be some type of
insurance. There are many companies offering insurance to cover the
eventuality that supervised aeromedical transport becomes necessary.
Many of the programs are directed toward large groups in the corporate
system. The expense and logistics of selling programs to individuals are
burdensome. Individuals normally only consider purchasing such insurance if a risk has been made apparent.

The cost of servicing aeromedical operations is high. With limited
enrollment of subscribers, this makes for a relatively high annual pre-
mium which is hard to relate to the chances of benefit. Those made
aware of the enormous expense of long-distance aeromedical evacuations, such as when an individual has been required to personally finance
a mission, may see the cost of premiums in a reasonable light. The need
for air evacuation insurance is not as apparent to most as is the need for
insurance against fire, theft, or hospital costs.

Wider Access

The need for improving access to aeromedical care deserves a wider
approach than just considering the needs of single individuals. This
country, and the rest of the world, is being plagued with more and more
disaster situations. Aircraft have demonstrated their value in many of the
operations required to meet the disasters. The performance of helicopters in the rescue of many persons from the MGM Hotel in Las Vegas
and the dramatic display over the Potomac River in Washington D. C.
when an airliner crashed into a bridge demonstrated the need for aeromedical services. At many of the newsworthy disasters, aircraft somehow
appear. However, the appearances, in most cases, were fortuitous, without being planned for in a logical way. There is no nationwide organization or service readily available to cover those areas where disaster may
strike. Disaster strikes every few minutes on lonely highways at points
not in easy reach of hospitals by ground ambulances. Only a few fortu-
nate communities have helicopter rescue services for the severe trauma
victims on the highways way out of town.

How to Improve Access

Some nations, notably Germany, have addressed the problem and have nationwide aeromedical rescue and evacuation services. They are sometimes financed by a large number of individuals, modest contributions entitling access to the services. The services can also be contracted to municipalities or legislative regions on a term basis rather than for fees related to specific service missions. Such financing underwrites expensive international aeromedical evacuations and allows humanitarian missions to other countries suffering disasters.

Plans are afoot for such an organization in the United States, and its realization should open access to aeromedical care for many who could benefit from it. It is expected that the air ambulance and rescue services already operating with satisfactory standards will be available on a mission contract basis to the nationwide, nonprofit organization. A national organization could never cost-effectively own and operate sufficient aircraft, equipment, and bases to service the whole country. Present services would need some coordination.

Technology

Looking to the future of aeromedical transport from the point of view of technological advances, lessons may be learned from the N.A.S.A. Space Program, the container-transport business, and the advanced critical-care units. It can be imagined that in the future patients might be transported in self-contained hyperbaric modules. Modules are already made for the transport of patients requiring biological isolation. Future modules may incorporate the means to correctly oxygenate the blood extracorporeally and circulate it at the correct pressure, temperature, osmolality, pH, etc., purifying the venous return. Computerized ventilation might prevent pulmonary atelectasis and pneumothorax. Intracerebral pressure may be monitored and regulated automatically. Computerized chemical and electrical control of cardiac rhythm and pump force might be included. The single medical flight attendant practicing the art of aeromedical care may be replaced by a team of biological engineers, biochemists, plumbers, and electricians. Accompanying relatives might be dehydrated on embarkation and rehydrated on disembarkation (or beamed ahead).

The logical concern with priorities rarely keeps pace with the incredible advances made in medical technology. In the future, should a patient be transported in an advanced critical-care module, the aircraft chosen for transport may still not be entirely suitable for the mission, the pilot might not be allowed to land because of inadequate documents, and the team of technicians may well be airsick. The inhalation of oxygen through a pipe stem from a bladder-like vessel made ballooning to higher altitudes possible but not comfortable. Present aeromedical technology does permit the safe and comfortable transport of the ill and injured in the "not-so-wild blue yonder." The skies have been made somewhat more friendly.

Physicians, nurses, and paramedics who accept duty as medical flight attendants will find an interest and excitement that is guaranteed to produce a sense of achievement as they earn their wings in the waiting skies.

Index

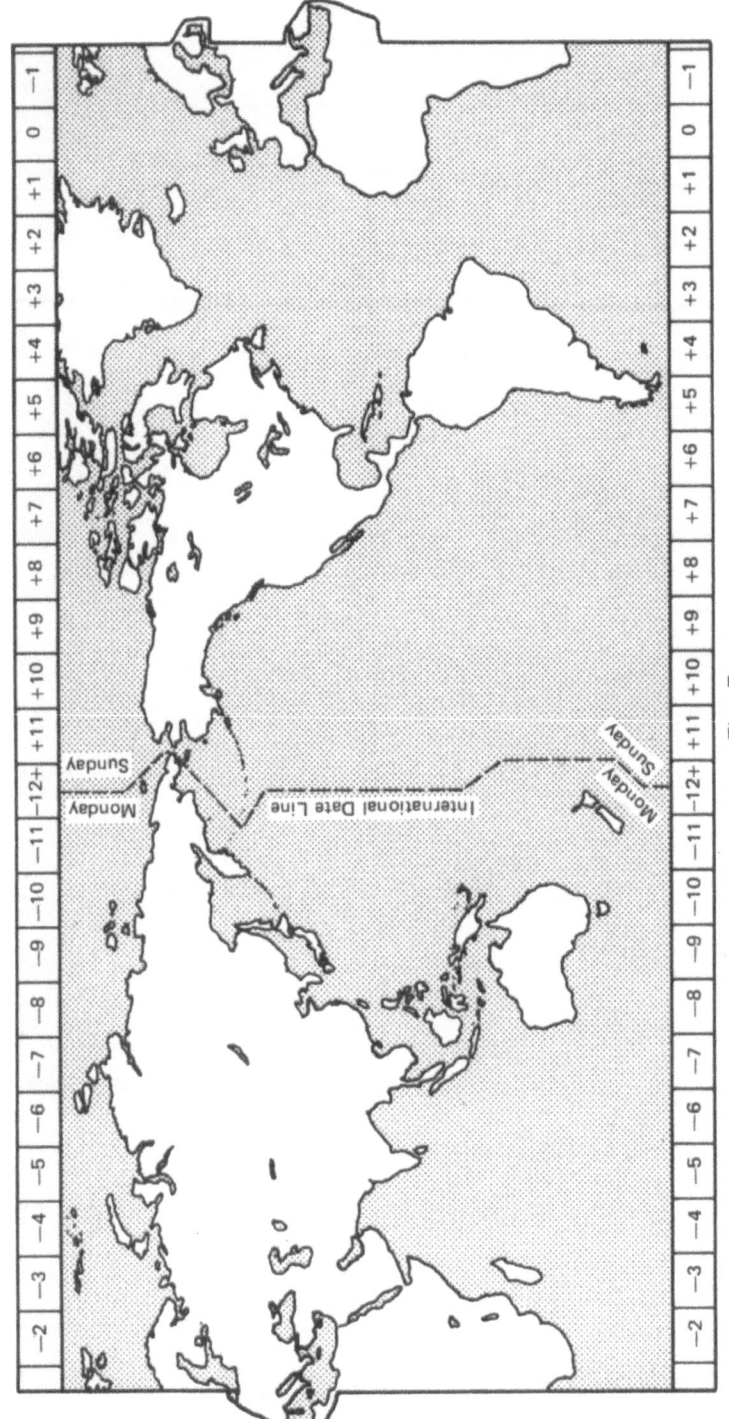

Time Zones